HELPING YOUR CHILD

CHILD

LOSE WEIGHT

THE HEALTHY

WAY

HELPING YOUR CHILD
LOSE WEIGHT
THE HEALTHY WAY

A Family Approach to Weight Control

Judith Levine, R.D., M.S.
and Linda Bine

CITADEL PRESS
Kensington Publishing Corp.
www.kensingtonbooks.com

CITADEL PRESS books are published by

Kensington Publishing Corp.
850 Third Avenue
New York, NY 10022

All Kensington titles, imprints, and distributed lines are available at special quantity discounts for bulk purchases for sales promotions, premiums, fund raising, educational, or institutional use. Special book excerpts or customized printings can also be created to fit specific needs. For details, write or phone the office of the Kensington special sales manager: Kensington Publishing Corp., 850 Third Avenue, New York, NY 10022, attn: Special Sales Department, phone 1-800-221-2647.

Citadel Press and the Citadel logo are trademarks of Kensington Publishing Corp.

First Kensington printing: December 2001

10 9 8 7 6 5 4 3 2 1

Printed in the United States of America

Library of Congress Control Number: 2001094205

ISBN 0–8065–2283–6

One of the luckiest things that can happen to you in life is ... to have a happy childhood.

—AGATHA CHRISTIE

In the effort to give good and comforting answers to the young questioners whom we love, we very often arrive at good and comforting answers for ourselves.

—RUTH GOODE

Contents

Part IV. Focus on Fitness

Part V. Facilitate Change

Part VI. Recipes

Acknowledgments

Thanks to Dr. Harry Coren, Child and Adolescent Psychiatrist, for sharing his expertise with us. His insight and knowledge about the psychological development of children were invaluable.

Thanks to Harry Somerfield for his ongoing support.

Thanks to our agent, Linda Allen, for never giving up.

To the Reader

WHY DID YOU PICK THIS BOOK off the shelf? Because you're a good parent, that's why. You're concerned that your six-year-old daughter never lost her baby fat. You're worried because your ten-year-old son has been gaining a lot of weight lately. You're upset because your thirteen-year-old daughter is always going on fad diets. You know you need to do something, but you don't know what to do.

You are not alone in your frustration. One in five children in the United States is overweight. Many of their parents are just like you—worried that their chubby child will grow up to be a fat adult. They understand the health risks of heart disease, stroke, diabetes, and the other serious illnesses that obesity contributes to.

You love your child. You don't want him or her to suffer the cruelty of taunting classmates, the frustration of failed diets, or the health hazards of becoming an obese adult.

We wrote this book for you and your chubby child because we're concerned about the physical and emotional health of all children. But we know that dieting doesn't work any better for children than it does for adults. So, instead of a diet, we will show you how to help your child grow out of his* extra weight, while building life-long, healthy attitudes about foods and fitness.

We'll share with you a variety of strategies for weight loss that won't stunt your child's growth or bruise her psyche. But it will be up to you to choose the solutions that address the specific needs of your child and are compatible with your family's lifestyle.

The book is divided into five parts. The first part will guide you through an assessment of the conditions that have an impact on your

---

*Instead of using phrases such as "his or her" or "he or she," we have elected to alternate the references to boys and girls, whenever possible. So, when you read a sentence that uses the pronoun "she," it doesn't indicate that the statement refers only to girls, and one with "he" doesn't refer just to boys. However, there are times when we will make specific comments about traits or patterns of boys compared to those of girls.

child's weight. Only by identifying the combination of factors that have contributed to his excess weight can you begin to change them. Through a series of questions about your child's behavior, family environment, physical development, and self-image, you will gather information to help him in a responsible and effective way.

In part II, you will learn how children are different from adults when it comes to weight control. For example, because growing children have different nutritional needs than adults do, it could be dangerous to put a child on an adult diet plan. Also, you will discover how, by making healthy changes in food and fitness, your child can grow out of her extra weight.

In part III, we will focus on food, exploring the different roles that parents and children should play in relation to food and eating. We will provide accurate information on how to put together a healthy, well-balanced, reduced-calorie eating plan for an overweight child. In addition, we will offer strategies, tailored to each age level, for influencing your child to make better food choices. Our approach involves gradually changing eating habits, encourages healthy snacking, but never eliminates favorite foods.

Part IV focuses on fitness, explaining the important role exercise plays in regulating a child's eating and body weight. The emphasis in this section is on encouraging physical activity that is fun, noncompetitive, and family-oriented. The child's age and interests are taken into consideration to help you increase your child's exercise level while decreasing his television viewing time.

In part V, we will help you with the process of making the changes that are necessary to help your child lose weight the healthy way. Depending upon your child's age and sensitivity about her weight, you will have to decide whether to involve her actively in the changes or if it would be better to be more subtle in your efforts. In this section, we will address ways to be supportive and nurturing of your child regardless of which methods you choose. Also, we will help you with ways to talk with your child about food and fitness, depending upon his or her age. And because of their increasing prevalence among children, we also will address such serious health risks as extreme obesity, anorexia, and bulimia.

As you read this book, and as you begin to try some of our suggestions, please keep in mind that your attempts to help your child achieve a healthier weight must be moderate and positive. By making moderate, gradual changes, you will ensure that your efforts will not harm your child in any way. Extreme measures not only are ineffective, they also can be unhealthy or even dangerous. Changes in eating and activity patterns have to be acceptable to your child or they simply won't work. While it's true that adults are able to punish themselves with strict diet and exercise regimes, children need a more positive approach. And finally, because the strategies we will teach you are moderate and positive, they can be integrated into your child's life and the lifestyle of your entire family. It's those kinds of changes that will help your chubby child grow up to be a fit and healthy adult.

PART I

First, Assess Your Child

1

Does Your Child Think He's Fat?

THIS IS A GUIDE FOR PARENTS. But the focus of the book isn't you, it's your child. You may already have thought about whether you should mention this book to your youngster, share some of the information with her, seek an active partnership, or just quietly make some positive changes she won't even notice.

You know your child better than anyone, but we would like to offer one suggestion: Please read the whole book yourself before you decide whether to show it to your offspring. You may feel that certain chapters would be appropriate to share with him or you may find it more effective (and less stressful) not to involve him overtly in your plans.

You're reading this book because you're worried about your child's weight. But before we discuss *your* concerns, let's focus on your *child*. What does your child think about his or her body?

A variety of factors can influence your child's body self-image, but probably the most important is what family members do and say. Certainly, if siblings tease him about being fat or his grandmother offers suggestions for losing weight, the message will be that something is wrong with him. This is likely to have a negative impact on the way he sees himself. And what family members *do* is as powerful as what they *say*. A study of fourth-graders found that children with family members who were on weight-loss diets were very likely to think they needed to lose weight, too. This was true for overweight children as well as for those youngsters whose weight was normal.

People in your child's life outside of the family also have an impact on her self-image: Comments from teachers, classmates, and friends help shape her body image. And, of course, the role models she sees on television—lean-bodied athletes, curvy movie stars, and pencil-thin fashion models—influence her perceptions of herself.

Has your daughter ever talked to you about being dissatisfied with her body? Has she ever made negative comments about her size or weight? Your chubby child may not come right out and say, "I think I'm fat," but she's probably sent you some indirect messages in what she says or does. It's not hard to tune into these messages. Do any of the following scenarios sound familiar? If so, your child may already be worrying about her weight or body size.

One day, ten-year-old Cheryl is dancing around the house, excited about trying out for a part in the school play, A Chorus Line. A couple of days later, she drags home from school, despondent because she didn't get picked as a member of the "chorus line," even though her two best friends did. That night, she eats only salad and vegetables for dinner—a real change from her usual hungry appetite. While she helps her mother with the dishes, she keeps talking about the play and how she wishes she were like Michele, who got picked for the lead part. "She's so pretty and popular," Cheryl laments. She stops short of saying "I wish I were thin like Michele," but her mother gets the message that Cheryl thinks she didn't get picked for the play because she's fat.

Fourteen-year-old Trevor used to like sports, but since he put on some extra weight last summer, the picture has changed. When he comes home from school, he's upset because he didn't make it onto the junior varsity football team. "The coach said I can't run fast enough to be on the team," he wails. "He had us run around the field and I came in last every time. I felt like such a dork." His father understands that Trevor's extra weight is keeping him from enjoying sports activities.

When her mother wants to take six-year-old Marjorie shopping for some new summer clothes, Marjorie says she doesn't feel like going to the mall. Instead they go to a neighborhood store. Marjorie fusses about having her mother in the dressing room with her, and gets very upset when her mom opens the door when she has all her clothes off. She quickly covers herself up and turns her back to the door. She doesn't like any of the outfits her mother picks out. Finally, she's reasonably happy with a pair of baggy pants and an oversized T-shirt. Her mother gets the idea that Marjorie is embarrassed to have her mother, or anyone else, see what her body looks like.

What Your Child Says ...

Your child may be sending you some pretty clear messages about how she feels about her weight and body. As she stands in front of the mirror, does she earnestly ask, "Mom, am I fat?" Has your son ever come racing into the house crying, "Mickey called me a fatso. Make him stop." Have you ever taken your daughter shopping and had her say, "Mom, this bathing suit makes my stomach look fat." Or, after she eats a special treat like birthday cake, does she ask if she looks fat because she knows that cake is fattening? Has your son ever talked to you about what he eats or told you that he wants to be on a diet? Do any of these comments sound familiar? If so, your child probably would be open to the idea of working on controlling his or her weight.

Or, your child may be sending you more subtle messages. Your daughter might compare herself to skinny friends, famous models, or actresses and athletes who are thin. Or, she may make comments like, "I wish I had legs like Andrea's." Is she envious of a classmate who's more popular with boys—and who also happens to wear a size three?

You might hear your son complain that he can't keep up with his friends when they go bike riding up the hills in the park. Is he spending more time playing video games alone in his room instead of being outside with his buddies?

Does your daughter come home from a friend's sleepover, upset with herself for pigging out on fattening food all night?

If these scenarios ring true, your child probably does believe she is overweight. She may be sending these messages, hoping that you will ask her more about how she feels. Try to use your child's comments about food and her body to gently broach the subject. In chapter 23, we'll share some suggestions on how you might do this.

What Your Child Does ...

Often actions speak louder than words. Your child may not *say* anything to indicate that he thinks he's fat, but he may behave in ways that give you some strong indications.

Have you noticed changes in your child's eating patterns that look suspiciously like "dieting"? Has she skipped meals? Has he asked for half a portion instead of his usual seconds? Did she refuse her favorite dessert? Did he say he didn't want to stop for pizza after the game? Will she now drink only diet sodas? Does he insist on using artificial sweetener on his cereal?

What about clothes? Does he wear "tent"-type clothes to cover his stomach? Does she wear a T-shirt over her bathing suit when she goes in the water? Does he make it clear that he doesn't want anyone to see him without clothes on—even his parents? Does she try in vain to squeeze into the "skinny" skirts all her friends are wearing?

Maybe he decided to give up a favorite team sport, or has refused to play games, such as relay races, at birthday parties or family picnics? Does she weigh herself every day? Twice a day?

When you notice one of these behaviors, it might be a good opportunity to ask in a loving way about the thoughts and emotions behind the actions. It might serve as a good opportunity to open communication on the subject and talk about how she really feels about her body image.

Is Your Child Ready to Slim Down?

Because a parent's view of a child has the greatest impact on how she feels about herself, you have to be very careful how you approach your youngster about her weight. It may be best to be completely open and honest about it, or it might be better to be more subtle. You will have to assess whether it's better to target strategies to work on alone (or with the help of your spouse) or whether it would be appropriate to involve your child as a partner in the project.

Chances are your child's situation resembles one of the following five cases.

1. *It's clear that he's troubled about being overweight and wants your help in slimming down.* If you've already discussed the subject and he's comfortable with the idea, you can actively involve him in many of the strategies we will suggest. But you will still have to decide whether to tell him that the suggestions come from this book. Remember, it was written for adults, not children. So, even if your child is interested in playing an active role in his weight control, we

don't generally advise letting him read the book. It will be best if you interpret the information for your child. Or, if he's old enough, you might carefully choose a few pages or a chapter to read together.

2. *She thinks she is overweight, but she has her own ideas about how to lose weight.* Some of her ideas may be too restrictive or nutritionally unsound. You may be able to help her accept less harmful ways to work on her weight by being a partner in the effort.

Again, you will have to decide the relative merits of letting her know that you are reading a book to help her with her weight. Seriously consider whether showing your child the book could trigger her to rebel by either drastically restricting her food or by overeating. If, on the other hand, you think that letting her know about the book will demonstrate that you're making a sincere effort to help her with her problem, you may want to do so. Maybe your child will be more likely to accept the advice from a book than from you. The bottom line: If you have any doubts, keep the book to yourself.

3. *She thinks she's overweight, but isn't motivated to do anything about it, or she's very touchy about the subject and gets upset at any mention of her weight.* When the doctor mentions her weight, does she ignore his comments? Does she complain that the kids at school call her names, but then dismiss it by making a flip comment?

4. *He doesn't think he's overweight, but you think he is.* If he hasn't said anything directly or indirectly, and he hasn't exhibited any of the "dieting" behaviors we mentioned, it's very possible he doesn't worry about his weight. If so, he probably won't be motivated to work on changing something he doesn't see as a problem.

If your child is somewhere between number three and number four, he's not ready to work on his weight. So, don't push it—you might make matters worse. But don't worry, we will teach you many subtle, gradual changes you can make in your family's eating and activity habits that will help your child without his even noticing it. In some ways, this approach may be easier because it averts potential confrontations, providing you can make modest changes and keep things low-key.

5. *Your child thinks she's overweight, but she really isn't; or she's very concerned that she's going to get fat.* In either case, you can use techniques in this book to teach her how to feel more secure about her body. This will help to avoid potentially more serious distortions

in her body image, which could lead to eating disorders, such as anorexia and bulimia.

As you continue reading this book, always keep your child's feelings and perceptions in mind. It's okay if they're different than yours, as long as you recognize the differences and try to understand his point of view. His attitude about his body will play a vital role in which slimming strategies you choose and how you talk to him about them.

And all along the way, we'll help you not only with issues of eating and exercise, but also with attitudes about food, fitness, and body image—both your attitudes and your child's. You see, knowledge, attitude, and behavior are all interconnected and thus influence one another. So, we will not only provide you with the factual information you need to make changes, we will also help you and your child develop positive attitudes. Both are essential to helping your child lose weight the healthy way.

When it comes to developing lifelong, healthy habits, starting early is one of the keys to success. So, keep reading.

2

Is Your Child Overweight?

SO YOU'VE DECIDED THAT your child is overweight. Is it something you've had a feeling about for a long time, or is it a more recent notion? Are you finding that her pants are getting too tight before they're becoming too short for her? Did you just have to buy jeans that were two sizes bigger than his last pair? Is she chubbier than her sister was at the exact same age? Has a well-meaning relative commented on how chunky he's getting? Does it seem to you that she's eating more than she needs? Did you son's doctor say on the last visit that he gained more weight this time than last time?

Even if all of the above are true, it doesn't necessarily mean that your child has a weight problem. A more objective way to begin to assess your child's weight status is with growth charts—the same tools that physicians use to determine how a child is growing.

Keep in mind, however, that using the charts is not the only way to assess a child's weight status, but it is a good place to start. In the chapters that follow, we will suggest that you gather a variety of information to help put together a complete picture of your child's unique growth pattern.

Measuring Your Child

The first step in using the growth charts is to accurately measure and weigh your child. If this was done quite recently at the doctor's office, you might call and ask for the measurements. Otherwise, you can weigh and measure your child yourself.

To accurately measure height, have your daughter stand in her bare feet, as straight as possible, with her head, back, and heels up against a wall or door frame. Be sure that her knees are not bent and that her heels are not lifted from the floor. Place a lightweight, rigid, flat object, such as a wooden ruler or hardbound book, on her head. Be sure it's resting flat on her head, parallel to the floor. Where the bottom of the book or ruler touches the wall, make a mark. Then use a tape measure or yardstick to determine the distance between the floor and the mark you made. Record her height in inches—you might even write it on the wall, along with the date. Kids love to see how they're growing.

As for weight, your bathroom scale is fine. It's best to weigh your child in his underwear, in the morning, before breakfast. After all, you want to weigh him—not his clothes and food. And for consistency, when you need to check his weight again, do it the same way and at the same time of day. This includes using the same scale, because every scale weighs slightly differently.

Calculating BMI

Although there are a number of different types of growth charts, ones that are based on body mass index have become the standard for pediatricians, dietitians, and other health professionals.

Body mass index (BMI) is a number that expresses the relationship between an individual's height and weight. The greater a person's weight compared to their height, the higher their BMI will be.

At every age, there is a range of possible weights and heights for "normal" boys and girls and, therefore, a range of possible BMIs. To figure your child's BMI, do the following calculation. (For accuracy, set your calculator to register at least four numbers to the right of the decimal point.)

_____ ÷ _____ ÷ _____ × 703 = _____

Weight in pounds ÷ height in inches ÷ height in inches × 703 = BMI

Here is an example of this calculation for a child who weighs 90 pounds and is 56 inches tall.

90 ÷ 56 = 1.6071
1.6071 ÷ 56 = .0286
.0286 × 703 = 20.175 . . . rounded off to a BMI of 20

Using the Growth Charts

The next step is to plot your child's BMI on the appropriate CDC Growth Chart for your child's gender. For a daughter, turn to the blank BMI chart on page 14. Along the bottom, find her age—in full or half years.

The BMI numbers are displayed on the right and left sides of the chart. So, if a girl is 12 years old and has a BMI of 18, you would follow the line straight up from the number 12 at the bottom of the page, and then follow the line that runs horizontally from the number 18 at the left or right of the page—to find the point where they intersect. (See the sample on page 13.)

Each chart also has a set of curved lines with corresponding labels (5th, 10th, 25th, 50th, 75th, 85th, 90th, and 95th) called percentile curves. The percentiles are based on the average growth of children nationwide. So, from where we placed the "X," follow the curved line to the right side of the page—you'll see that she's at the 50th percentile for BMI. This means that 50 percent of children her age have BMIs higher than hers and 50 percent of them have BMIs lower.

What Do the Numbers Mean?

While most children fall between the 25th and 75th percentiles, a child whose measurements fall outside of these ranges for her age is likely to be completely normal, too. For example, a child in the 20th percentile may not be getting a diet that is nutritious enough to provide for proper growth. Or, she might be just naturally very slender. Likewise, a child who is at the 80th percentile could have a weight problem, but perhaps he's just getting ready for a big growth spurt. This is why we say growth charts cannot be used alone. They must be interpreted in the context of a child's life and balanced with factors such as eating patterns, exercise, and family history.

However, according to health experts, a BMI at or above 85 percent indicates that your child is probably overweight—the higher the BMI, the more likely there is a problem. Although a onetime assessment of a child's BMI, can point to a potential weight problem, another way to use the growth charts is to plot a child's BMI over time. Patterns will become more apparent and one-time spikes will be put into perspective.

For example, if a child is at the 60th percentile for BMI at age 3, and is at the 75th percentile by 4 years old, the parent might be concerned that she is gaining weight too quickly. But, when her BMI is back to the 65th percentile at age 5, the parent would see that her growth adjusted on its own. On the other hand, if by 5, she were at the 85th percentile, you'd see a pattern emerging that might need attention.

Putting the Numbers in Context

If you or your child's doctor has a record of his or her height and weight for the past couple of years, you can calculate the corresponding BMIs and plot them according to your child's age at the time the measurements were taken. When you look back, you may see that your son's BMI percentile for his age stayed about the same until last year—when it jumped to a much higher level. This jump in weight may be the start of a new pattern, or it could be a onetime blip in a normal growth curve.

In any case, if your child is experiencing a deviation from his previous growth pattern and seems to be gaining more weight than height, consider whether anything unusual has been going on in his life recently. Perhaps the weight gain is due to a reduction in physical activity, or maybe he's been eating more as a way to cope with a new stress in his life. Did he quit little league? Has he been glued to his computer day and night? Has he been upset by something happening at home or in school? If you can't explain the "out of proportion" weight gain in terms of a special occurrence, maybe it's simply because he is getting ready for a growth spurt.

In any event, the advice in this book will help you teach your child how to keep a healthy weight for the rest of his or her life. Learning good eating habits at an early age is the best prevention for obesity and the most reliable predictor for a long-term maintenance of a normal weight.

Sample BMI Chart for Girls

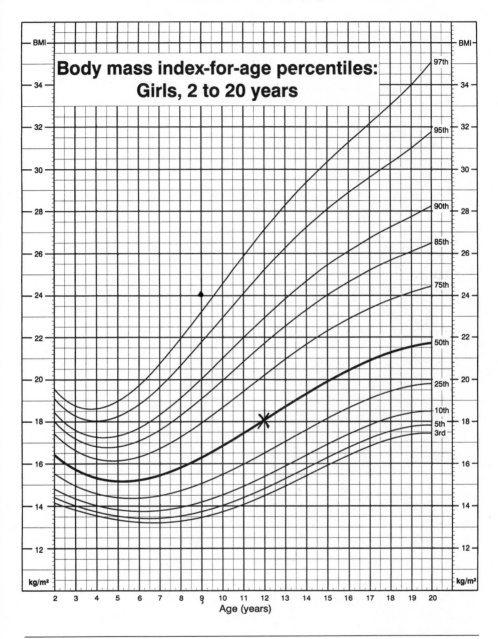

Body mass index-for-age percentiles: Girls, 2 to 20 years

Source: Developed by the National Center for Health Statistics in collaboration with the National Center for Chronic Disease Prevention and Health Promotion (2000): divisions of the Centers for Disease Control (CDC).

13

Blank BMI Chart for Girls

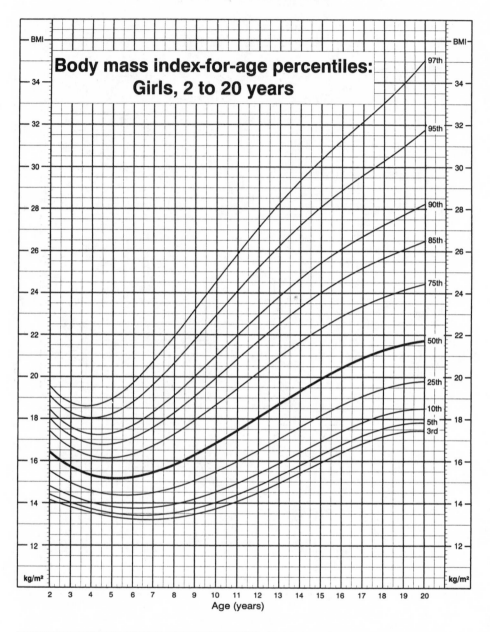

Body mass index-for-age percentiles: Girls, 2 to 20 years

Source: Developed by the National Center for Health Statistics in collaboration with the National Center for Chronic Disease Prevention and Health Promotion (2000): divisions of the Centers for Disease Control (CDC).

14

Blank BMI Chart for Boys

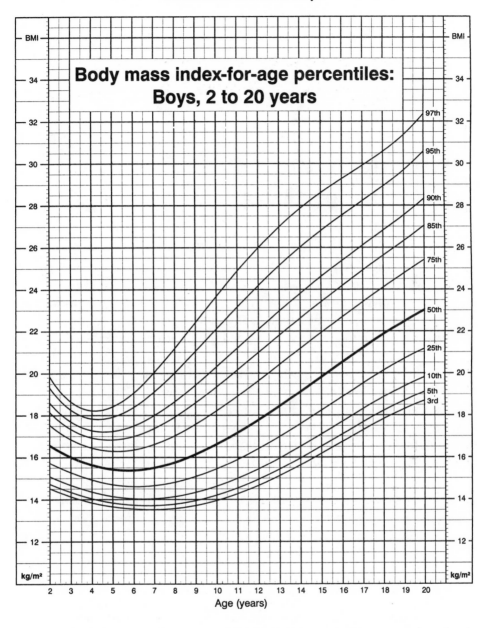

**Body mass index-for-age percentiles:
Boys, 2 to 20 years**

Source: Developed by the National Center for Health Statistics in collaboration with the National Center for Chronic Disease Prevention and Health Promotion (2000): divisions of the Centers for Disease Control (CDC).

15

3

Are Mom and Dad Overweight?

A CHILD IS A REFLECTION OF her mother and father and maybe even other members of the family. She has her father's red hair, her mother's brown eyes, her grandfather's disposition, and her grandmother's sweet tooth. In the same way, a child inherits from her family a variety of factors that influence her height and weight and body shape. Therefore, as part of determining whether or not your youngster has a weight problem, it's important to consider her heredity.

Heredity has a significant influence on a child's weight. Although there is a lot of variation on an individual basis, a number of scientific studies suggest that if both parents are obese, a child has an 80 percent chance of being obese. If only one parent is obese, the child's risk is closer to 40 percent; and if neither is obese, there is perhaps a 10 percent likelihood that the child will be. These studies looked at how adopted children resembled their biological parents more than they did their adoptive parents. So, it's clear that a child can inherit the tendency to be overweight.

This tendency may be affected by one of several potentially inheritable factors, including metabolism and body composition.

- *Metabolism.* A person with a relatively slow metabolism burns fewer calories than someone with a faster metabolism. Therefore, inheriting a slower metabolism can make a child gain weight more easily and make it harder for her to lose it.

- *Body composition.* Some people are more prone to respond to excess calories by gaining fat, while others tend to gain muscle. A child who inherits the propensity for gaining fat rather than muscle is more likely to become obese.

But this doesn't mean that a child with overweight parents is doomed to be a chubby child or a fat adult. However, when exposed to certain environmental influences, a youngster who has inherited the same biological factors that make his father and mother overweight will be more likely to become overweight himself than a child who doesn't have this genetic handicap.

How Genetics Influences a Child's Weight

It's similar to the situation of having two children in a family who inherit different complexions. The red-haired, fair-skinned girl has a greater likelihood of getting sunburned than her olive-complected, dark-haired brother—but only if she's exposed to too much sun. The catch is that the amount of sun it takes to give her a bad burn is not likely to affect her brother at all; it would take a great deal more exposure for him to get sunburned. The girl can protect herself from getting burned by using sunscreen and wearing a hat, while her brother doesn't need to bother.

Say the tables are turned with regard to their predisposition to becoming overweight. If the boy inherited the tendency to be chubby, but his sister did not, it may be much harder for him to keep from becoming overweight. A lot will depend upon their family's eating and activity habits. And just as she has to use sunscreen to keep from getting burned, he may have to indulge in junk food less often and exercise more often to keep from getting fat.

This is not a hypothetical situation. It is a sad truth that two children in the same family can eat the same amount of food and one will become overweight while the other will stay slim. Unless they are identical twins, two siblings may have very different genetic makeups.

One way to demonstrate genetic influences on weight is to study different sets of identical twins. That is exactly what one group of researchers did. For more than three months, they purposely overfed twelve pairs of identical-twin, young-adult males. They were fed 1,000 more calories per day than they needed. At the end of the time period, each young man had gained approximately the same amount of weight as his twin. Both of them even put on the weight in the same parts of their bodies: Some twin pairs tended to develop spare tires around their middles, while others gained most of the weight in their hips and thighs.

But as important as the fact that identical twins gained weight similarly was the finding that each pair gained differently than the other pairs. In fact, one pair gained about ten pounds, while another gained nearly thirty pounds. All of the men in the study were assigned equal amounts of moderate physical activity, so exercise did not account for these differences in weight gain. The researchers also found that some of the pairs of twins put on most of the weight as fat and others gained more muscle than fat.

The study illustrates that while genetics is a strong underlying factor, it is still just one factor: The researchers had to feed the young men 6,000 extra calories a week—equivalent to six pints of gourmet ice cream—and restrict their activity in order to make them gain these significant amounts of weight. Indeed, a variety of fat-promoting behaviors can and do override genetic tendencies.

Children Inherit More Than Your Genes

In a less biological way, your child can "inherit" your eating and exercise habits. You may be unaware that you are a role model of behaviors that your children can pick up. Children usually do as you do, in spite of what you may say. Do any of these fat habits sound familiar?

- Do you put butter on everything?
- Do you eat mostly meat and potatoes—rarely chicken, fish, or vegetables?
- Do you eat candy bars as regular snacks?
- Do you insist on dessert at every meal?
- Do you pig out when you eat out?
- Are second helpings automatic?
- Do you belong to the "clean plate club"?
- Are you a fast eater?

- Do you eat in front of the TV?
- Are you unable to watch TV without snacking?
- Do you always buy candy and popcorn at the movies?
- Do you reach for food every time you're stressed out?
- Do you eat just because you're bored?
- Do you spend hours surfing the Internet?
- Do you choose TV over outdoor activities?
- Do you consider exercise a chore?
- Do you always take the car to do neighborhood errands?
- Do you take elevators instead of the stairs?

If you answered "yes" to more than a few of these questions, you are likely to be contributing to your child's chubbiness.

Your Child's Future Outlook

What does your child's genetic picture look like? Is Mom overweight? Does Dad weigh more than he should? If you answered "yes" to both questions, does that mean that your children are destined to be overweight too?

The answer is "no, not necessarily." Although the genetic influence is real, it is not the only predictor of a child's future weight. If both parents are overweight, there is a strong likelihood that without intervention their child will be an overweight adult. However, making appropriate changes in diet and exercise at a young age can totally change the outcome. In fact, positive behavior changes that children make seem to be more effective than similar efforts by adults, in part because they haven't had the bad habits as long as the grown-ups have. That's one of the most important reasons to help your child adopt healthy habits at an *early* age.

Also, there is some evidence that a true genetic predisposition to fatness, as opposed to "inherited" habits that contribute to obesity, can be most effectively overcome with exercise. This may be because exercise can help speed up a metabolism that has a hereditary tendency to be slow. So if both of your chubby child's parents are obese, you may want to pay particular attention to the exercise chapters in this book.

What if only one of you is overweight and the other is at a healthy weight? It will be harder to predict how much influence each of your genetics will have on your child. But because she may take after the parent who is overweight, it's prudent to take preventive measures as early as you can.

If both of you are at a healthy weight, there is less of a chance that your child will grow up to be an overweight adult. However, if he seems chubby to you now, you shouldn't ignore the fact and just assume that he will grow out of it. Although you are both thin, your child's eating and activity behaviors could override his favorable genetics. Continue with the other assessment chapters to identify factors that may be affecting your child's weight.

4

What, When, Where, and Why Does Your Child Eat?

WHEN YOUR CHILD was a baby, you knew about every morsel of food she ate and every ounce of fluid she drank. And now that she's older, you may think you still know exactly what she eats and drinks. But, chances are, you may not know as much as you think. Do either of these examples sound familiar?

Four-year-old Sam has breakfast at home before his father drops him off at the day care center. The center provides his morning and afternoon snacks, so his parents don't know what he eats then. And even though his mother packs his lunch box, his parents don't really know what he eats for lunch either. He may gobble up everything, or he may dump his carrot sticks. Maybe he'll trade his sandwich for a cupcake. And even when Sam is at home, it's hard for them to be certain what he eats. His father may know that he gave Sam animal crackers and milk for a mid-morning snack, but he has no idea that Sam also got some chips from his older sister or drank half of his brother's soda before lunch.

Or what about ten-year-old Sarah? Although she fixes her own breakfast, her mother is there to see that it's a bowl of cereal or a bagel and milk—not a soda with a handful of cookies. But Sarah buys her lunch at school and comes home after school with her older brother. She has full access to the kitchen until her mother gets home. And to complicate matters further, Sarah spends every other weekend with her father and stepmother. Her mom has no idea what she's eating there.

So how can you get an accurate picture of your child's eating patterns? And why should you bother?

We'll answer the second question first. The purpose of this book is to help you devise a plan that is tailored specifically to help your child slim down. There is no generic eating plan that is appropriate for every child, or every chubby child—one size does not fit all. What will work for Joseph might not be the right strategy for Joanne. A cookie-cutter approach just doesn't cut it.

Throughout the book, we will be offering suggestions and ideas to help address a wide variety of issues and problems that affect chubby children. The good news is that not *all* of these problems will apply to your child. It's up to you to pick the strategies that address the specific needs of your youngster. But before you can look at solutions, you have to assess the problems. That's why it's important to look objectively at your child's eating patterns, to help pinpoint opportunities for improvement.

How can you do this? We've provided two tools for you: a Food Record and an Eating Behavior Survey. By completing the Food Record as thoroughly as possible and answering the questions accurately, you will have a much more objective picture of what, when, where, and why your child eats.

Food Record and Eating Behavior Survey

You don't eat the same food in the same way every day and neither does your child. His eating behavior varies from day to day. In order to get as complete a picture as possible of your child's eating patterns, we suggest that you fill out the Food Records for four consecutive days—two weekend days and two weekdays. Complete the record as soon as possible after he eats. At least do it on the same day: If you wait, you're apt to forget something.

We're going to ask for a lot of detailed information. Remember, it's just for four days, so try to be as complete as possible. These details will be especially helpful as we get into problem solving later in the book.

What your child eats is not just a question of type of food, it's also how the food is prepared and how much of it your child consumes.

When your child eats is important as part of the assessment, too. For example, you might find that he's not eating anything between lunch and dinner. Maybe that's why he's ravenous at dinner and tends to overeat.

Where your child eats can influence food intake as well. If you record that your daughter eats all of her snacks in front of the television, maybe you'll come to realize that watching TV is a trigger for her eating.

Why your child eats may sound obvious, but sometimes children, like adults, eat for emotional reasons rather than because they are physically hungry. Anger, boredom, and stress can trigger eating— even with children.

As you read on, you will learn even more about the importance of pinpointing what, when, where, and why your child eats. You will see that each aspect of eating has the potential for creating problems and that each requires a different kind of solution.

The Food Record and the Eating Behavior Survey are not designed to pass judgment on you or your child. Their only purpose is to collect objective information.

When you complete the Food Records, try to fill in as much information as you can without involving other people or drawing attention to the assessment. If the subject of food (and weight) is highly sensitive to your child, don't ask her about what she ate, just do your best and fill in what you know. However, if you're doing this as a joint project, go ahead and ask your daughter about meals and snacks you didn't see, such as a school lunch bought or a snack at a friend's house. And, if necessary, enlist the aid of the day care provider.

Write in the *time* your child ate breakfast, lunch, and dinner, as well as snacks between meals. If it's more than one snack, write the time for each snack.

Write *where* your child ate the food. This includes the location in your house (kitchen, bedroom, dining room, TV room) as well as where he ate outside of your house (at school, at day care, at a restaurant). If you know that he ate dinner at a friend's house, just write the location and time. You won't know what he ate unless he mentions it.

Also include comments that will help you recall special circumstances or observations, such as "Dad's birthday," or "had seconds," or "didn't like the beans." You can also comment about why you think your child ate, or that he was "starving" when he came to dinner.

Food and Beverages

This is the heart of the Food Record. Be as specific and complete as possible. If he didn't eat a meal, write "none" in this column. If you don't know what he ate for a meal, write "don't know."

Breakfast

- If it's "cereal," indicate what kind and what type of milk was on it—fat free, reduced fat (1% or 2%), or whole. Try to estimate how much cereal she took. Did she add more cereal later to use up the leftover milk in the bowl? Figure that into the quantity. Was there fruit on the cereal? What kind?
- Be detailed about things like toast. White or whole wheat? One piece or two? Was it buttered? With jelly? Both?
- Don't just write "juice." Say what kind and approximately how many ounces.
- What about other beverages, such as milk or hot chocolate?

Did we forget anything?

Lunch

- Don't just put "sandwich." Note that it was a tuna sandwich made with oil-packed tuna and regular mayonnaise on French bread. Mention if there was additional mayonnaise on the bread, too.
- If it's a turkey sandwich, was there cheese on it? What kind of cheese? Was there mayonnaise or mustard or butter on the bread? What about lettuce and tomato?
- Was the sandwich toasted or grilled?
- Did he eat chips? Was it a handful? Or more?
- Did he have a piece of fruit? What kind? How much?
- Were there cookies? How many? What kind?
- What did he drink? Soda? Milk? Juice?

Are you getting the idea?

Dinner

- With salad, include what vegetables went into the salad and what kind of dressing you used.
- If it's "chicken," indicate how it was cooked and which piece she ate. If it was a leg, did she eat two? Did she eat the skin?
- Was the rice steamed or fried?
- Don't just put "potato." Say French fries. If it was a baked potato, did she eat it with butter or sour cream? Or both?
- Don't just say "pasta." Put what kind of sauce was on it: tomato, cream, pesto?
- Write "broccoli," but also note if there was butter or cheese sauce on top.
- Dessert? What type, how much? Did the Jell-O have whipped cream on top? Were there second helpings of ice cream?
- Don't forget the extras, such as bread and butter, olives, or pickles.

Got the hang of it?

Snacks

A snack is what your child eats between organized meals. The amount of food and the time may vary. It may be an apple at mid-morning, or a few crackers and cheese or a candy bar after school. It could also be a bowl of popcorn while watching an after-dinner movie. Just for these four days, keep track of it all, as best you can.

Be a Detective

As we said, compiling an accurate Food Record is not always easy. It may take a bit of detective work. Here are a few suggestions for sleuthing out the facts, or for working with just a few clues.

Lunch Box Queries

Does your child make his own school lunch? If so, try to observe as he's packing it. Do you make his lunch? You know what you sent, but how do you know that he ate it? If you can't ask him, just write down what you sent. If it's a lunch box instead of a lunch bag, check the returned box for uneaten food. What about trades? Maybe there will be evidence of unfamiliar wrappers that come home in the box.

Slippery Snacks

Once a child is old enough to help herself to snacks, it's hard to always know when she snacks and what she takes. On the four days you're doing the Food Records, try to hang around and observe as much as possible.

Day Care Dilemma

If your child goes to day care for all or part of the day, talk to the day care provider and ask her to cooperate with your Food Record by filling in as much as she can for you. Ask her to be discreet and not involve your child.

Food at Friends' Houses

You won't know what your child has eaten if he spends time at a friend's house. You might be able to casually ask him. But if not, simply write "don't know" by a specific meal he ate away from home.

Joint Custody Quandary

If your child spends most weekends with her father, you will have a major gap in the Food Record. If she goes there more than twice a month, consider asking him for some assistance. Remember to explain to him if it's important that your daughter not be involved in the Food Record. If your relationship with him isn't cordial, just skip it and record two weekend days your daughter spends with you or do four weekdays instead.

To get you started, here are a couple of sample Food Records. They are followed by a blank one for you to photocopy to use for your child.

Food Record for: Jennifer (age 16)

Date: ___March 13_____   Day of the Week: ___Thursday_____

	Time	Food and Beverages	Location	Comments
Breakfast	7:30 am	apple	at bus stop	in a rush, late for school
Snack(s)		don't know		
Lunch	12:30 pm (5th period)	ham & cheese sandwich on hard roll with mayo. small bag of chips 8oz. box of orange juice	at school	this is what she packed in her lunch this morning, may have bought something else at school
Snack(s)	3:30 pm (after school)	big bowl of ice cream 2 Oreo cookies	kitchen	said she was "starving"
Dinner	6:30 pm	2 pieces of fried chicken (leg & breast with skin) mashed potatoes with gravy (2 servings) water to drink	kitchen	skipped the spinach
Snack(s)	9:00 pm 10:00 pm	handful of chocolate chip cookies (4–5) can of soda (orange)	watching TV	homework done

Food Record for: Michael (8 years)

Date: _____ October 10 _____   Day of the Week: _____ Saturday _____

	Time	Food and Beverages	Location	Comments
Breakfast	7:30 am	chocolate puff cereal with whole milk	kitchen	helps himself
Snack(s)	10:00 am	4 snack crackers and 1 slice of American cheese 1 glass apple juice	family room	hungry
Lunch	noon	peanut butter & jelly sandwich on white bread handful of potato chips glass of grape juice 2 chocolate chip cookies	kitchen	he's in a peanut butter & jelly rut
Snack(s)	3:00 pm 4:00 pm	2 cups of apple juice ice cream cone— one scoop	at soccer practice in car	stopped on way home from practice
Dinner	6:30 pm	½ bowl of spaghetti with meat sauce 1 piece of bread with butter 1 glass of whole milk 2 chocolate chip cookies	kitchen	didn't want all of his spaghetti but insisted on dessert
Snack(s)	8:30 pm	bowl of microwave popcorn (shared bag with sister) 1 cup of grape juice	living room	watching TV

Food Record for: _____

Date _____ Day of the Week: _____

	Time	Food and Beverages	Location	Comments
Breakfast				
Snack(s)				
Lunch				
Snack(s)				
Dinner				
Snack(s)				

Eating Behavior Survey

This part of the assessment asks you to think about a variety of issues that relate to your child's behavior in relation to food. This will help you to consider more than just the food itself. Don't judge your child or yourself as you address these issues; just try to be as accurate and complete as possible. Your honest observations are vital if you are going to come up with solutions to help your child lose weight the healthy way.

Why does your child eat? Does he/she eat . . .	Never	Sometimes	Often	Always
when truly hungry?				
when bored?				
when tired?				
when under pressure?				
when angry?				
when upset?				
when sad?				
because friends are eating too?				
when there are too many tempting foods around?				

How does your child eat? Does he/she . . .	Never	Sometimes	Often	Always
eat fast?				
eat slow?				
gobble up the food so he/she can go out to play?				
savor every bite of food?				
ask for second helpings?				
prefer snacks to meals?				
want to eat when someone else in the house is eating?				

What does your child eat? Does he/she . . .	Never	Sometimes	Often	Always
turn up his/her nose at any new food?				
love all food?				
throw a fit if he/she doesn't get chips? dessert? soda?				
eat cookies first and fruit only when there are no cookies in the house?				

When does your child eat? Does he/she . . .	Never	Sometimes	Often	Always
eat 3 meals a day?				
skip any meals?				
want a snack right after a meal?				
snack all day long?				

How do you interact with him/her about food?	Never	Sometimes	Often	Always
Are there "food rewards" for good behavior?				
Is "no dessert" used as a punishment?				
Does he/she have to sit at the table until the dinner plate is clean?				
Does he/she have to eat every bite of dinner to get dessert?				

All of the information that you've gathered will be invaluable when you get to chapters later in the book that offer suggestions and solutions to common problems. There's no point working on problems that your child doesn't have. You want to implement suggestions that address his or her specific needs. By really understanding your child's eating and activity behaviors, you will be able to choose the solutions that will work best for him or her.

5

Is Your Child
Physically Active?

Max spends Monday through Friday working behind a desk. He gets no physical exercise other than walking from his house to the bus stop. On weekends, he spends hours sprawled on the couch watching TV, often snacking on sodas, potato chips, and sweets. Sound like the portrait of the typical American male? Well, what about the typical American boy?

Recent studies reveal that millions of parents are actually more physically active than their children. We have the illusion that kids spend a lot of time running around playing, but in reality, many of them are lured into inactivity by television, video games, and other high-tech, sedentary distractions.

On average, two- to five-year-olds watch television four hours a day, and six- to eleven-year-olds watch TV three and a half hours daily. The more time a child spends in front of the TV, the greater the chance that he or she will be overweight. Watching television is a triple whammy, contributing to weight gain because (1) it doesn't take much energy to watch, (2) it keeps a child away from more physical activities, and (3) it is often accompanied by snacking on high-calorie foods.

Kids want to have fun, but exercise sounds like work. The most important factor determining whether a child will engage in a physical activity is if she enjoys doing it. The second most important factor is her parents—whether they exercise themselves, provide opportunities for her to exercise, and generally encourage her to be active.

Everyone knows that food is related to weight, but did you know that physical activity is probably even more important when it comes to preventing and controlling childhood obesity? A study of a group of infants showed that the fattest babies ate the least and were also the least active. The leanest babies were the most active and ate the most. A study of teenage girls also supports this relationship: The overweight girls tended to eat less than normal-weight girls, but also were much less active.

Exercise offers important benefits to weight control for children:

- It burns calories.
- It can increase metabolism.
- It helps control appetite.
- It can build muscle, which helps burn fat.
- It can improve a child's sense of well-being.

But exercise doesn't have to be in the form of an organized fitness program or competitive sport in order to provide many of these benefits. Activities such as walking to school, playing catch, or roller-skating are better for improving fitness than being a couch potato.

Your Exercise Attitudes and Behaviors

Since parents are so influential in determining whether a child is physically active, we would like you to think for a moment about your own exercise attitudes and behaviors. What you believe, say, and do can have a profound effect on whether your child gets enough exercise. How many of the items on the Activity Encouraging List on page 35 sound like you? What about the Activity Discouraging List?

A Tale of Two Ten-Year-Olds

A child's attitudes and behaviors about exercise and other physical activities are the result of heredity, natural abilities, and family influences. Take a look at the differences between Lucy and Samantha, two fifth-graders in the same school.

Activity Encouraging Attitudes and Behaviors of Parents	Activity Discouraging Attitudes and Behaviors of Parents
Limit the time a child can watch TV and play video games	Allow the child to watch TV, as long as homework is done
Reward a child with fun, physical activity	Reward a child with TV watching or use TV as a baby-sitter
Include the child in physical activities the parents enjoy doing	Get exercise only alone or with other adults
"Let" the child win at a game sometimes	Always play competitively, even with young children
Spend a sunny afternoon outside doing something physical	Spend a sunny afternoon at the movies
Enjoy exercise, or at least make an effort to do some every week	Don't exercise and don't hide the fact that they hate to exercise
Plan weekend outings or vacations that are active	Plan weekend outings or vacations that involve mostly driving or sitting

Lucy spends a lot of time in her room. When she's not studying, she's either talking on the phone to her friends or watching TV with her sister. Favorite outings with her friends are either going to the movies or going shopping. Although it's only about a mile to the mall, she gets her father to drive her, unless he's glued to the television watching a ball game. She takes after her mother when it comes to being klutzy, so she isn't good at sports. Since physical education isn't required in fifth grade, she takes an art class instead. She isn't lazy. She helps her mom with the cooking. The family usually eats dinner in the kitchen, watching the news on TV. Lucy really enjoyed her family's vacation at the lake last year. She spent hours lying in the sun reading books, but refused to take off her beach cover-up and go in the water.

Samantha isn't hyperactive, she just doesn't like to sit still. Her mother says she's antsy. She rushes through dinner so she can go outside and play. She walks to school with her brother and takes gymnastics after school on Tuesdays and Thursdays. On the weekend, she usually goes in-line skating with her friends in the neighborhood or for a bike ride with her mom and dad. She likes sit-coms on TV, but her mother will let her watch only for an hour after her homework is finished. Her family went on a backpacking trip over spring break and Samantha had a great time learning to kayak.

Who do you think is more likely to have a weight problem—Lucy or Samantha?

Well, now it's time to focus on the exercise attitudes and behaviors of *your* child. The following Activity Assessment will help you get a clearer picture of how physically active or inactive your child is. Because of the importance of family habits, some of the questions also ask about family activity patterns. We'll look even more closely at family dynamics in the Family Favorites Chart later in this chapter.

As with the Food Record and Eating Behavior Survey in chapter 4, try to be as thorough as possible and answer the questions accurately. You will use this information in later chapters when we offer suggestions and strategies for boosting your child's activity level.

Activity Assessment

1. How much TV does your child watch in a week? How about other family members? _____

What is the weekly total of television watching for
    your child?   _____ hours

How much time a week does he/she spend:
    sleeping?   _____ hours
    lying down at rest?   _____ hours
    studying?   _____ hours
    playing video games or sitting at the computer?   _____ hours

2. Does he/she walk to school?   yes/no
    one way?   yes/no
    both ways?   yes/no
    how many days a week?   _____ days
    how far is it each way?   _____ blocks

3. Does he/she bike to school?   yes/no
   how many days a week?   ____ days
   how far is it each way?   ____ miles

4. Is there physical education at school?   yes/no
   how many days a week?   ____ days
   how much time is each class?   ____ minutes

5. Does he/she do organized after-school or weekend activities or sports?
   how often?   never / 1 day a week / 2 days / 3 days / 4 days / 5 days
   for how long each time?   ____ minutes

What sports? Check all that he/she has done in the past twelve months:
   ____ baseball/softball
   ____ T-ball
   ____ volleyball
   ____ football
   ____ tennis
   ____ basketball
   ____ hockey
   ____ rowing
   ____ soccer
   ____ swimming
   ____ other: _____

6. What classes has he/she taken in the past twelve months?
   ____ art
   ____ music
   ____ ballet
   ____ gymnastics
   ____ ice skating
   ____ martial arts—karate, tae kwon do
   ____ weight training
   ____ aerobics
   ____ swimming
   ____ other: _____

7. Does your preschooler's day care program offer an opportunity for physical exercise?
 none / very little / some / plenty

8. What kinds of weekend activities does your child do alone, with family or friends?

Activity	never	sometimes	often	all the time
Watching TV				
Sitting at the computer				
Playing video games				
Going to the movies				
Bowling				
Horseback riding				
Playing Ping-Pong				
Playing Frisbee				
Playing catch				
Playing hopscotch				
Hitting a tennis ball alone				
Skiing, downhill				
Social dancing				
Hiking/backpacking				
Tennis game				
Roller or in-line skating				
Ice skating				
Bicycling				
Skiing, cross-country				
Walking				
Swimming				
Jogging				
Jumping rope				
Other:				

9. Around-the-house activities?

Activity	never	sometimes	often	all the time
Walking the dog				
Folding laundry				
Dusting				
Doing the dishes				
Ironing				
Sweeping up				
Vacuuming				

10. Do you drive your child to school, to the movies, to his/her friend's house?

     always / often / sometimes / never

    Could he/she walk or ride his/her bike?

     never / sometimes / most of the time

    Is age or safety an issue?

     yes / no

It's a Family Affair

We talked about the important role parents play in determining a child's activity level, so we'd like you to consider what *you* do for fun. When you're not working or doing household chores, what are your favorite activities? What about your spouse?

And since a child's enjoyment of an activity in large part determines whether he will participate in it, we also want you to look at your youngster's preferences. This is somewhat different from the Activity Assessment because we're asking you to consider what your child enjoys doing most and least—which may be somewhat different from what she actually does on a daily or weekly basis. For example, she may love swimming, but can't do it very often because there's no swimming pool in your backyard. Or she may prefer to spend free time reading a magazine, but doesn't have much time to do it because of schoolwork and household chores.

Rate the following activities. Put a 1 by your absolute favorites, a 2 for those that you enjoy somewhat, a 3 by those that you would do only under special circumstances, and a 4 by those that you'd have to be dragged to kicking and screaming. Do the same for your child, or better yet, ask him about his favorites. Put a 1 for his top choices; a 2 for things he does enjoy, but not as much; a 3 for things he will participate in reluctantly; and a 4 for activities he never does or would refuse to do if given the choice. Put an "X" for those that do not apply, such as "working out at the gym" for a four-year-old, or "playing outside with friends" for Mom.

We'll look at this chart more closely in the later chapters dealing with suggestions for making fitness fun, and strategies for involving the whole family in activities that will help your child slim down. But this preview of the Family Favorites Chart may begin to reveal how much your child's activity choices mirror yours.

Do you find that most of your favorites and his are in the top half of the chart? Then chances are your preference for sedentary activities has been influencing your child. Do you have mostly "1s" and "2s" in the bottom half? Then, you're probably a pretty active family. If you seem to like more active pursuits than your child, you may need to plan more fun activities for the whole family. Another possibility is that your youngster takes after just one parent when it comes to his or her favorites.

In many ways, technological advances, such as automobiles, elevators, televisions, and computers have made life easier and more enjoyable for us and our children. But such inventions also have created lives that are perhaps too full of conveniences. Increasingly, our lives and our children's require minimal amounts of physical exertion. As a result, we and our children may have to make a special effort to get up off the couch, to get out from behind that desk, to get out of the car, and move! Remember, a little activity is better than no activity at all.

Family Favorites Chart

Activity	Child	Mom	Dad
Reading a book or magazine			
Going to the movies			
Talking on the telephone			
Taking a nap			
Baking a new recipe, or helping parent in the kitchen			
Going out to eat			
Watching TV			
Surfing the Internet, or e-mailing friends			
Playing video games			
Going for a ride in the car			
Going to the shopping mall			
Gardening or helping in the garden			
Going dancing			
Playing outside with friends			
Going hiking			
Going for a walk			
Bike riding/in-line skating			
Working out at the gym			
Snow sports			
Playing competitive sports			
Taking a class that's active			
Swimming			
Going jogging/running			

6

Can Your Child Grow Out of Her Weight?

"DON'T WORRY, SHE'LL GROW OUT OF IT." That's what doctors often tell the parents of a chubby child. But parents do worry, because what if their child doesn't grow out of his or her extra weight? All too often, this extra weight stays extra. To help keep this from happening, the advice we offer in later chapters will show you how to use your child's future growth to the greatest advantage.

Children grow continuously. The most rapid growth occurs during the first four years of life. The other major increase in height takes place during what's referred to as the adolescent growth spurt. For girls this usually happens between ten and fourteen; for boys it's generally later, between twelve and sixteen. However, in between these two periods of especially rapid growth, a child continues to grow every year, though at a less dramatic pace. This is good news for you and your child, because you can take advantage of both the steady growth of early and middle childhood and the growth spurt of adolescence to help your youngster grow out of any extra weight.

The following chart shows the average yearly height increases for boys and girls of average height for their age. Although these numbers do not reflect the number of inches your child has been growing or is going to grow, they will give you some idea of the continuous nature of growth throughout childhood and adolescence. The chart demonstrates that boys and girls grow at much the same rate until puberty. And it also shows the differences between boys and girls as they enter and go through puberty. Girls start and end their adolescent growth spurt earlier than boys do. This gives boys the advantage of a couple of more years of growth before puberty, one of the major reasons that boys generally grow to be taller than girls.

How Children Grow
Average Height Increases in Inches

Year	Boys	Girls
1	10.0	9.0
2	4.5	4.5
3	3.5	3.5
4	3.0	3.0
5	2.5	2.5
6	2.5	2.5
7	2.5	2.5
8	2.5	2.5
9	2.2	2.2
10	2.5	2.3
11	2.0	2.7
12	2.5	2.5
13	2.7	2.2
14	3.0	1.5
15	2.5	0.8
16	1.7	0.3
17	0.5	0.0

There are six questions to consider when trying to answer the question, "Can my child grow out of his or her weight?"

- How overweight is your child?
- How old is your child?
- Are his or her parents overweight?
- How tall are his or her parents?
- Has he or she started puberty; if so, when?
- Are you ready to make some family changes to help your youngster eat better and be more physically active?

Weight

In chapter 2, you plotted your child's BMI on the growth chart to determine the percentile for his or her age. As we discussed, if your child's BMI percentile is 85% or above, she probably is overweight. The higher the percentile, the more certain you can be that she is overweight. And the more overweight your child is, the less likely it is that she will grow out of her extra weight without some type of intervention. However, with changes in eating and exercise habits, it can be done, especially if she has some time left to grow.

Age

The earlier you can help your child with her eating habits, the greater the advantage growth will provide in helping her to slim down. A girl who is five years old has between nine and eleven more years to grow; a five-year-old boy has between eleven and thirteen years of growing time left. In this length of time, you can help your child make gradual changes in eating and activity patterns that can help to assure that he will grow out of his weight.

At ten, the girl has just four to six more years to grow, while the boy has six to eight years. A teenager has even fewer years of potential growth left, although boys still have more than girls. For both boys and girls, these years will be decreased further if a child goes through puberty early or especially quickly.

Helping a younger child grow out of his weight is easier than trying to help an adolescent, because a younger child has more years and, therefore, more inches to grow. But that's not the only reason. You're better able to influence the food choices of a younger child, and he is more likely to listen to your advice and follow your role modeling than a teenager is. As children grow up, they start assuming greater responsibility for the food they eat. They eat more meals away from home and they have money to buy snacks of their own choosing. Also, it's difficult for parents to limit the sedentary activities of teenagers and encourage more active ones. That's not to say that you can't help a teenager slim down, it's just that you'll have to use different strategies than with a younger child.

Parental Weight

Studies have shown that if one or both parents are significantly over-weight, there is a greater risk that their children will grow up to be overweight adults. This is especially true for children under ten, even if the child is not currently overweight.

What this suggests is that if you and/or your spouse are over-weight, it would be wise to begin changing the family's eating and exercise patterns as soon as possible—even if you're not sure that your child is overweight. Not only will it help you reduce your own risk of weight-related diseases, it will likely turn the tide for your overweight child, and help keep a normal-weight child from growing into an overweight adult.

Parental Height

The next question is, "How much more is your child going to grow?" The only definitive way to know is by x-raying her wrist. This is not a routine part of a visit to the doctor—these kinds of x-ray studies are used only for children who are suspected of having growth prob-lems, such as a deficiency of growth hormone.

A more practical way to make a general prediction about a child's adult height is to look at her parents' heights. The chart on page 46 is designed to use the average of the parents' heights to predict the approximate adult heights of their children. However, because of vari-ations, such as when a child goes through puberty and how long that phase lasts, this prediction is not exact.

We'll take you through the process, step-by-step.

Step 1. How tall is Mom in inches?
    Example: Doris Jones is 5 feet 4 inches or 64 inches.
Step 2. Convert Mom's height to centimeters by multiplying inches by 2.54 (centimeters per inch).
    Example: $64 \times 2.54 = 162.56$ (round off to 162.6 centimeters).
Step 3. How tall is Dad in inches?
    Example: Ed Jones is 5 feet 10 inches or 70 inches.
Step 4. Convert Dad's height to centimeters.
    Example: $70 \times 2.54 = 177.80$ (177.8 centimeters).

Step 5. Average the two heights by adding them together and dividing by two. This number is the Midparent Stature.

Example: 162.6
          +177.8
          340.4 ÷ 2 = 170.2 cm

Step 6. The chart indicates the predicted height at age eighteen for a boy and a girl for a variety of Midparent Statures. Look at the number corresponding to the Midparent Stature of a child to estimate his or her height at age eighteen.

Example: Adam Jones (Ed and Doris's son) could grow to be between 176.2 and 180.5 centimeters. So, let's say his growth potential is approximately 178 centimeters.

Step 7. Convert centimeters back to inches by dividing by 2.54.

Example: 178 cm ÷ 2.54 = 70.1 inches or 5 feet 10 inches

Step 8. Subtract the child's current height from his potential height, based on Midparent Stature, to get an estimate of how many more inches he may grow.

Example: Adam is 5 feet tall now, so 5 feet 10 inches − 5 feet = 10 inches more to grow, potentially.

Possible Height—Based on Midparent Stature*		
Midparent Stature in Centimeters	Potential Height of a Girl at Age 18 in Centimeters	Potential Height of a Boy at Age 18 in Centimeters
161	156.2	not applicable
163	161.0	171.5
165	165.0	175.0
167	167.2	177.9
169	164.3	176.2
171	164.4	180.5
173	167.9	180.2
175	171.8	178.6
177	165.7	177.6
178	170.8	186.3

*Adapted from Garn, S.M., and C.G. Rohmann. Interaction of nutrition and genetics in the timing of growth and development. *Pediatr. Clin. N. Am.* 1966; 13:353.

Now, let's consider Adam's sister, Megan.

The 170 cm Midparent Stature for girls shows a predicted adult height of 164.3 to 164.4—or approximately 164 cm. When we convert centimeters to inches we get 64.5 or 5 feet 4½ inches. Since Megan is currently 5 feet tall, she has perhaps 4½ inches left to grow.

Now, figure out the Midparent Stature for your child and calculate his or her possible growth potential.

Step 1. How tall is Mom in inches? _____ inches

Step 2. Convert Mom's height to centimeters by multiplying inches by 2.54 (centimeters per inch).

_____ in. × 2.54 = _____ cm. Round off to one decimal point _____.___ cm.

Step 3. How tall is Dad in inches? _____ inches.

Step 4. Convert Dad's height to centimeters.

___ in. × 2.54 = _____ cm. Round off to one decimal point _____.___ cm.

Step 5. Average the two heights by adding them together and dividing by two. This number is the Midparent Stature.

Mom's height   _____ cm

Dad's height + _____ cm

_____ cm ÷ 2 = _____ (Midparent Stature)

Step 6. Look at the line for this Midparent Stature, or the one closest to it, and write down the potential height for your son or daughter at age 18.

_____ cm

Step 7. Convert centimeters back to inches by dividing by 2.54 to get your child's potential height in inches.

_____ cm ÷ 2.54 = _____ inches

Step 8. Subtract your child's current height from his potential, based on Midparent Stature.

Child's potential height   _____ inches

Child's current height   – _____ inches

Potential additional growth _____ inches

Puberty

The age at which a child goes through puberty greatly influences his or her adult height. In fact, it is one of the reasons the Midparent

Stature is a less-than-perfect predictor of a child's adult height. The age at which a given child begins puberty is genetically determined, as is the length of time it takes her to complete this transformation to adulthood. Both variables have a profound influence on an individual's adult height.

A girl who begins the process of puberty at ten years old is likely to start menstruating at twelve. After the onset of menstruation, she has perhaps two to three more years of moderate growth left. A girl who doesn't start menstruating until she's fourteen has two extra years of growth and is likely to be taller when she finishes growing than the girl with the earlier onset of puberty. Also, a girl who completes puberty in two years is more likely to be shorter than a girl who takes four years to go through the whole process.

In boys, puberty begins later than in girls. This gives boys the advantage of more years to grow before that final spurt. You can see from the chart on page 43 that the average boy might grow five inches between fourteen and seventeen, while the average girl gains only about an inch during those years.

Putting It All Together

The five factors we've been discussing—a child's age, her degree of overweight, her parent's weight status, her potential adult height, and her status with regard to puberty—are independent variables that influence the ability of a chubby child to grow out of her extra weight. To see how these variables fit together, let's look at three different children.

Juliette is 4 years old. She's 37 inches tall, and at 33 pounds, her BMI is 17. This puts her a bit above the 85th percentile for her age. She has approximately 10 years before she finishes her adolescent growth spurt, and based on her parents' heights, she could grow as much as 28 more inches. Juliette has plenty of time and not too serious a weight problem . . . yet. She's in an excellent position to grow out of her weight, with some consistent help with food and exercise. However, because her parents are both overweight, the whole family needs to start now to make significant lifestyle changes. Otherwise, Juliette could grow up to be an overweight adult, like her mom and dad.

At 6 years old, Bruce is 44 inches tall and weighs 50 pounds. His BMI is 18, which is above the 90th percentile. Bruce is considerably overweight for his height—but time is still on his side. His Midparent Stature indicates that he may have 23 more inches to grow in the 10 years before he is likely to finish puberty and neither of his parents is overweight. But the fact that Bruce is more than just a little chubby suggests that he may already have some eating and activity habits that are contributing to his being overweight. It's important to start changing those now. Perhaps he can even lose a little weight before he begins puberty.

Vickie is 14 years old. She's 5 feet 4 inches tall. At 135 pounds, her BMI is 23, which puts her around the 85th percentile for her age. This does prompt some concern, especially since she started menstruating when she was 12, and may have just a year or so more to grow. Her Midparent Stature indicates that she's likely to grow to 5 feet 5 inches. The issue with Vickie is that she doesn't have much growth left to take advantage of. But every little bit helps. If, over the next year, she can lose a little weight and grow a little more, that will put her closer to a healthy weight. Then, with the better eating and activity habits she will have learned, she can continue to lose a little more weight if she needs to—after she's finished growing.

As you read about Juliette, Bruce and Vickie, did one of them sound familiar? Well, now it's time to record the following information about your child:

1. Age: _____
2. BMI percentile: _____
3. Are one or both parents overweight? _____
4. Potential additional growth (from page 47): _____
5. Has he/she started puberty? _____ If yes, how long ago? _____

These are independent variables that can influence how easy or how challenging it will be to help your child grow out of his weight. There is no precise way to interpret the impact they will have individually or together on the likelihood that your child will grow out of his weight. But are you willing to take the chance that it will happen by itself?

Which takes us back to the last question we asked at the beginning of this chapter: Are you ready to make some family changes to help your child eat better and be more physically active? Because that's the only predictable way to help your child grow out of his or her extra weight.

7

How Does the Family Picture Affect Your Child?

FAMILIES COME IN ALL SHAPES AND SIZES: small, large; one-parent, two-parent; extended families; blended families; yours, mine, and ours. They live in cities, in suburbs, and in the country. For better or for worse, children are the products of their family environment. A child doesn't get overweight all by himself and he will not be able to slim down without the support of his entire family.

This isn't to say that a child's mother or father or other family members are to blame for his weight problem. Yet there is no denying the strong impact that family dynamics exert on a child's attitudes and behaviors relating to food and physical activity. While the influence of heredity on weight and body shape cannot be ignored, the *behaviors* a child "inherits" from his family are just as powerful as the genes he inherits—maybe even more so.

If your child is overweight, any family member who isn't part of the solution is part of the problem. This may seem blunt, but research studies demonstrate that family support for a child's positive changes in eating and exercise is vital to the success of her weight control effort. In fact, the most successful long-term results are achieved when parents and other family members participate in these lifestyle changes. Conversely, an uninterested or uninvolved family increases the likelihood that an overweight child will not be successful in slimming down.

In order to reveal ways in which you and the other members of your family can help your child attain a healthy weight, you need to stop and look at your family's food and fitness dynamics. In this chapter, we'll ask you to take a few "snapshots" of your family and also to look at some pictures of families that may resemble yours. You'll see that words and actions are meaningful features of these family portraits. Some of them are quite subtle—they lurk in the shadows or hide under good intentions. So you will have to look carefully at all the "pictures" in the family album to get the whole effect.

Family Features

Where does your chubby child fit into the family portrait? How many people are in her immediate family? Is she the oldest, the youngest, or in the middle? Is she an only child? Is she a preschooler, a grade schooler, a preteen, or a teenager? Do both of her parents work? It's interesting to note that research on the subject has found that mothers who work outside of the home provide meals that are just as nutritious as those prepared by mothers who don't. They do, however, feel more stressed and have less time for meal preparation.

Is there an adult at home when your child gets home from school? Maybe an older brother or sister baby-sits until a parent gets home. Who makes the rules about TV, meals, snacks? Who enforces the rules?

The answers to these questions begin to fill in the background of your child's family portrait. By themselves, these aspects of your child's life do not reveal anything significant about how his family influences him, but as we continue to paint the portrait, they may cast a shadow or highlight an emerging pattern.

Take a Home Tour

A home is more than a collection of rooms. Whether it's a sprawling ranch-style house or a tiny apartment, the contents and layout of a home influence the behavior of its inhabitants. For example, one research study demonstrated that, in general, girls were more likely to be physically active if there was exercise equipment around the house. And certainly the food that is brought into the home has an impact on what a child eats.

To visualize nine-year-old Mary's home, let's pretend we're looking at a video that takes us through the various rooms. The most prominent feature in the living room is the television. The couch and all the chairs are grouped around it. On the coffee table are the remnants of potato chips and dip, a few empty soda cans, and a half-empty bowl of peanuts. As we move into the kitchen, we see a box of candy on the table and a glass jar full of chocolate chip cookies next to the TV on the kitchen counter. Also on the counter top are a variety of appliances—a food processor, blender, breadmaker, pasta machine, and microwave oven. We look in the refrigerator. It's quite full of all types of food. In the vegetable bin there is a bunch of carrots, a head of lettuce, and some celery—all unwashed. In the freezer there are two half-gallon cartons of ice cream and a variety of frozen dinners. Moving on to Mary's room, we see a couple of snack wrappers and soda cans in the trash. On her desk is her own small TV and a computer.

Now let's go across the street and see how thirteen-year-old David's home compares. The front hall is a little cluttered with two bicycles, a pair of in-line skates, and a couple of tennis rackets. In the living room, we see a television in the corner, with an exercise bike pointed toward the screen. In the kitchen, there's a bowl of fruit on the table and a small jar of jellybeans on the counter. In the refrigerator we see a variety of foods, but prominent on the middle shelf is a container of carrot sticks, ready to eat, as well as a washed bunch of grapes. The freezer has some cans of orange juice, a carton of frozen yogurt, frozen vegetables, and a frozen pizza. David's bedroom is pretty typical for a teenager. It's hard to see anything but a blizzard of clothes, music tapes, and school books. But as we look around, we find a basketball, a skateboard, and a Frisbee. A pair of swim goggles hangs over the doorknob.

Did you pick up some clues to the food and fitness habits of these two families? If someone took a video of your house today, what would it reveal?

What's in Your Shopping Cart?

Although some children eat lunches provided by their school, and older children may buy some of the food they eat, the majority of your child's food passes through your shopping cart before it makes it to his plate.

Who does the grocery shopping in your family? Is it always Mom? Do Mom and Dad trade off, or is Dad the main shopper? Do you each buy different kinds of things when marketing? Maybe your child comes with you to the store. Does he ask you to get specific foods when you are at the market? What kinds of food does he request?

How often do you go shopping? Do you have to go every day to keep up with your hungry family? Do they seem to gobble up the goodies as fast as you can buy them? Or do you do one big trip each week? Maybe you stock up only once a month and then fill in with perishable items as needed in between. Does shopping for large-quantity bargains result in a lot more food around the house—which seems to disappear just as quickly as smaller quantities?

What kinds of food items are in your shopping cart? Try keeping track of your food shopping for a week. How many items purchased fall into each of the following categories?

Breads, cereals, grains? _____
Vegetables? _____
Fruits? _____
Meats, poultry, fish, and beans? _____
Milk and milk products? _____
Extras?_____
(Extras are treats, such as chips, cookies, candy, ice cream, soft drinks, fruit drinks, and other items, like butter/margarine, oil, mayonnaise, salad dressing, sour cream, sugar, sauces, condiments.)

As we will discuss in detail in chapter 12, when we climb the food pyramid, the daily recommendations for children include: six to eleven servings of breads, cereals, and grains; three to five servings of vegetables; two to four servings of fruits; two to three servings of meats, poultry, fish, or beans; and two to three servings of milk or milk products. Extras should be just that—served in small, limited quantities.

There are no specific goals for how many items from each category of food you should have in your shopping cart, but you get the idea. So how did your shopping cart measure up?

Someone's in the Kitchen

Who's in charge of meal preparation? Mom? Dad? Mom and Dad? Is the family cook a gourmet chef, or does he aspire to be? Does the cook do it out of necessity, relieved to get dinner on the table? Either extreme can create a less-than-ideal situation for a chubby child. The gourmet chef can spell trouble for a youngster who is especially motivated to eat when she is presented with particularly delectable food. And the cook who's more interested in speed than nutrition can end up serving fast, high-calorie food. In later chapters, we'll provide tips for gourmet chefs, reluctant chefs, and all the cooks who fall in between.

Other variables to consider include:

Do any of the children in the family help with the cooking? How about your chubby child?
Who makes breakfast and lunch?
Does the baby-sitter fix dinner and prepare the food her way?
Is there an avid baker in the house?

Look at Mealtime Through a Child's Eyes

A lot more goes on at a meal than just eating food. The dinner table, especially, is a place where family dynamics are played out. To get an idea of how mealtimes can affect a child, we're going to look in on three different children at dinnertime. Can you figure out which mealtime environment is least likely to contribute to a child's being overweight?

In Zachary's family, dinner is served at 6:15 P.M.—sharp! Everyone is expected to be in their seats on time, with hands washed. Mom already has salad plates at each place. Family members tend to eat their salad quickly, while Mom finishes cooking the rest of the dinner. She brings the individual dinner plates to the table, already served. The serving dishes go on the table for second helpings. The rules are straightforward and strictly enforced. Rule 1: Everyone is expected to eat everything on their plates. Zachary has spent more than one night at the table alone trying to finish a slice of cold meatloaf. Rule 2: If you don't eat all of your dinner, you don't get dessert. Conversation at the table seems like a string of orders: "Jeffrey, get your elbows off the table." "Zachary, watch out, you're going to spill your milk." "Don't talk with your mouth full." "Eat your beans."

At Sandra's house, dinner isn't tied to any particular time or place. It could be a sandwich in front of the TV at 6:00 P.M., a three-course meal in the dining room at 7:00 P.M., or a bowl of cereal in the kitchen at 8:30 P.M. Depending upon the time dinner is served, and what is served for dinner, a variety of snacks may or may not be available before or after the meal. In addition to a lack of predictability about timing and what is going to be served for dinner, there's no consistency about whether the family eats together or not. Dad may want to watch "Monday Night Football," while Sandra and her mother eat in the kitchen. Or Mom may have to work late, so Dad will stop on the way home for take-out.

At Dan's house, dinner is served consistently between 6:00 P.M. and 7:00 P.M. The family doesn't usually eat breakfast together, so they make a real effort to sit down together for dinner. Occasionally, the whole family will watch a special television program while eating dinner. But, usually, dinner is seen as a time to catch up on the day's activities. Dan and his sister, Deanna, are encouraged to join in the conversation. In fact, their parents make a point of asking their thoughts on topics of discussion. Mom does most of the cooking, but Dad is in charge of the salad, and Dan and Deanna take turns setting the table and clearing the dishes. The serving dishes are put on the table and everyone is able to take as little or as much as they want. The only rule is that a new food has to be at least tasted. If the children don't like it, they don't have to eat it.

Did you pick up any clues that would help you guess whether Zachary, Sandra, or Dan might be chubby? Studies indicate that the behaviors exhibited in Dan's home are the least likely to foster obesity in children. These include having the child help with preparing the food or setting the table; allowing him to make decisions about what he eats; giving small portions when introducing special or new foods; and encouraging the child to try a few bites of an unfamiliar food.

The dinner habits in Zachary and Sandra's homes are more likely to contribute to a child's weight problems. The over-controlling environment in Zachary's home can contribute to a child's being unable to learn on his own how to regulate the amount of food that is appropriate for his body. There was no opportunity for Zachary to choose the foods or the quantity of food he wanted, unless it was for seconds. Although having predictable times for family meals promotes healthy eating, being too structured can result in forcing children to eat when they're not hungry or have had enough. The other extreme, as exhibited in Sandra's home, is just as difficult for a child. Not knowing what to expect for dinner can cause a child to overeat snacks while waiting for the meal.

Other mealtime behaviors that can be detrimental to healthy eating include: putting too much food on the table; eating too fast; expressing displeasure if a child doesn't eat the food you prepare; restricting the food you serve to your child, while not limiting the food of other members of the family; and using dinnertime to solve difficult issues.

Certainly, it's the parents' responsibility to meet their children's nutritional requirements at meals, but they also should try to establish a positive and supportive eating environment so that the youngster can develop healthy food-related attitudes and behaviors. Mealtime should be a pleasant, enjoyable, relaxing time for everyone.

What About Eating Out?

For some people, eating out is a special treat; for others it is a frequent necessity. How often do you and your children eat a meal that isn't prepared in your kitchen? How often do you stop at fast-food places? What about eating at restaurants? What kind of restaurants do you usually pick?

If eating out is more than a rare event, it has a major impact on your family's eating habits. Luckily, restaurants of all types offer items that taste good and are good for you. In chapter 17, we'll help you learn how to make healthy choices when eating away from home.

Families Do More Than Eat Together

So far we've focused mostly on issues pertaining to family food behaviors: what type of food is purchased, who prepares and serves it, when and where it is eaten, and what kind of family interaction takes place around these food-related activities. Now we want to take a look at how your family members interact with one another when food isn't the main focus.

Is yours a supportive family where family members try to help one another? Do the kids stick together? Or is it more competitive, with each one trying to outdo the others in various activities and achievements? Are there rivalries? Are you judgmental toward your children, always expecting them to do better? Do the older kids pick on the younger ones?

Does your family spend a lot of time together, or do you tend to split up? What do you do for fun? Is food always part of the fun? Is fun more likely to be an outdoor or an indoor activity?

Do you and your spouse stick together, agreeing on important rules in the family? Do you agree on issues related to food and exercise? Or do your kids end up caught in the middle between Mom and Dad's differing rules and attitudes with regard to television watching, snacking, candy, whether they can have second helpings? Or maybe your child is caught in the middle between you and your ex-husband or ex-wife with regard to these issues.

Perhaps you and your spouse come from different food backgrounds. For example, maybe in your family, food was simply nourishment, while in your spouse's family, food was a symbol of nurturing and love.

How are your children rewarded? With praise? Toys? Food? Is food used as a bribe for good behavior? How are your children punished? Do you use time-outs? Do you restrict TV/video privileges? Do you take away dessert?

Deep down in your heart, how do you feel about your child's being overweight? Do you love and accept your child even though he's overweight? Or do you feel uncomfortable about it and think, "If only he didn't eat so much, he'd be thin?" Even if you don't think you are showing your displeasure, anxiety, or frustration, your child may be picking up on these emotions. Children are amazingly aware of their parents' unspoken thoughts.

Keep these ideas in mind as you read, and, in part V, we'll go into more detail about family attitudes and support.

Emotional Impact of Change

If your child has recently been putting on weight, it could be the start of a growth spurt, as we'll see in chapter 8. But, maybe, it's the result of some upheaval in her life that has affected her deeply. Has she experienced an emotional upset that she may be trying to cope with by eating? Did her parents get divorced? Was there a death in the family? Has a parent been ill? Are there problems at school? Is there a new baby in the house? Maybe you have noticed a change in her eating patterns since this trauma.

Not only can these kinds of disturbances cause your child to ease her emotional pain by eating, they also may have influenced your shopping or cooking habits. If you've been affected by the upset, too, perhaps you've had less energy to cook. Are you buying more prepared foods or eating out more often than before? Is someone else doing the cooking?

Your Family Portrait

To get a clear picture of your family environment, take this lifestyle quiz.*

Do you and your family:

	NO	YES
Have regularly scheduled mealtimes?	____	____
Eat meals together most of the time?	____	____
Eat planned snacks, as opposed to "anytime" snacks?	____	____
Choose portion sizes appropriate to your needs?	____	____
Plan and prepare meals together?	____	____
Make a point not to miss or skip meals?	____	____
Try to make mealtimes pleasant?	____	____
Avoid being members of the "Clean-Plate Club"?	____	____
Make dinner last more than 15 minutes?	____	____
Eat only in designated areas of the house?	____	____
Store most food out of sight?	____	____
Make sure you're hungry when you eat?	____	____
Avoid using food to punish or reward?	____	____
Enjoy physical activities together regularly?	____	____

---

*Adapted from © 1992, The American Dietetic Association. *"If Your Child Is Overweight."* Used by permission.

Limit your TV viewing time?   ____   ____
Frequently have fun together without eating?   ____   ____

If you answered "yes" to most of these questions, you're probably doing fine. If not, there is room for improvement. We'll help you make some gradual, but effective changes.

PART II

Children Are Different

8

Don't Put Your Child on a Diet

WE'LL SAY IT AGAIN, for emphasis: "Don't put your child on a diet."

"Why not?" you may ask, "I go on diets all the time."

The truth is, diets don't work for children any better than they do for adults. And worse, they can cause considerable harm to a child's growth, health, psychological development, and ability to learn.

Most diets are designed to make a person lose weight. For adults, it's almost impossible to slim down without losing some pounds. But, as we've already said, your chubby child may not need to lose any weight. Many children can use their height to help them grow out of their extra weight.

The second feature of most diets is that they are of limited duration. One goes *on* a diet and then proceeds to go *off* it. This is exactly what we don't recommend for you or your child. The premise of our book is that the best way to slim down is for your child and your family to make gradual changes in eating and exercise—changes that will become a part of your life for the rest of your life.

And while we suggest that you modify the eating patterns of your whole family, there are some members who should not be included—anyone under two!

Two and Under—No, No!

When it comes to eating, babies know best. From birth until the age of two, there should be no attempt to restrict their food intake. It is up to the parents to provide appropriate nutrition, as recommended by their child's doctor, and to let the baby determine how much to eat.

During the first year of life outside of the womb, an infant grows more rapidly than at any other time in his life. By the end of his first year, the average baby has tripled his birth weight. Adequate nutrition during infancy is critical to support this rapid rate of growth. And it's not just growth in terms of weight and height that's important: The baby needs proper nutrition in order to finish the maturation of his brain, internal organs, bones, and other parts of his anatomy that you can't see from the outside.

Although babies can't talk, they give clear signals about when they're hungry and when they're full: They cry in a distinctive way when they need food and may turn their heads away or stop sucking when they've had enough. Since each baby is different, there is no set feeding pattern that fits every child. And even though you know your baby well, it's still hard to assess whether she is eating too much or too little. The doctor, or other health care provider, who weighs and measures your baby at regular intervals is the best person to help you accurately determine the adequacy of your child's diet. All reputable health professional organizations agree that fat, cholesterol, and calories should *not* be restricted for children under two years of age.

However, this doesn't keep some conscientious parents from trying to impose restrictive diets on their infants. Concern for a baby's chubby thighs and round bellies, or fear that a baby *might* become fat, has motivated some misguided parents to engage in feeding practices that are harmful to their little ones. There are case studies in the medical literature of parents who restricted the number of calories, reduced the percentage of calories from fat, withheld treats, or did not allow between-meal snacks for babies under two years of age. These practices led to a serious retardation in growth, called "failure to thrive," among these babies. The parents did not intend to nutritionally deprive their children, but that's exactly what they did. The diets of these children provided insufficient calories and nutrients to sustain normal growth, so they didn't grow in height or weight at the proper pace. Fortunately, when the babies' diets were improved, so did their growth.

The bottom line is this: If your child is under two, put this book away, at least until he's had his second birthday. If you still have concerns about his weight, read it then. If you got this book because your elder child is chubby, apply the information to him and the older members of the family, but leave his baby sister out of it. Remember, a baby is the perfect regulator of her own food. That is, her appetite generally reflects the needs of her body for proper growth and development. She should be fed when she's hungry, but not forced to finish the bottle or clean the plate.

Because babies have small stomachs with a limited capacity, they need to eat often. So don't restrict snacks. And since babies can't eat a large volume of food, even when broken up into a number of meals and snacks, the food they eat has to be packed with nutrition. It's important for them to get the most out of the volume that their little tummies can hold. For example, children who have progressed to drinking milk, but are still under two years of age, need to drink whole milk—not low-fat. Their rapidly growing bodies need all the calories and fat that whole milk provides.

Certainly, the physical consequences of restricting calories or nutrients in a baby are important concerns, but there also can be psychological implications. You don't want your child to feel deprived and hungry during the formative years of his psychological development. Such experiences can have a long-lasting negative impact on how he perceives who controls his food supply. Also, early struggles can cause food to become a focal point for struggles later in childhood, as well as throughout his life.

Family Fear of Fat

It's not uncommon for parents to be afraid that a chubby child will grow up to be a fat, unhappy, and unhealthy adult. The reality is that obesity increases the risk of developing heart disease, diabetes, high blood pressure, and other serious diseases. It is also true that, in our society, with its obsession with thinness, overweight people are discriminated against and even ridiculed. We've written this book, and you are reading it, because we all recognize that being obese is not desirable. But when a concern about a child's overweight becomes a fear of fat, that's not healthy, either.

Fear of fat can make parents do the wrong things, unintentionally. And while the fear may be justified—with a family history of obesity or an already overweight child—it's important that you don't over-react and compromise your child's growth or contribute to the development of an eating disorder. We'll help you walk the tightrope between prudent actions and harmful reactions.

Some parents' fear of fat is not grounded in reality. Sometimes adults are simply preoccupied with weight and fat. They may be compulsive exercisers and chronic dieters. They may be thin, but worry relentlessly about getting fat. Or they may engage in strict diet and exercise regimes sporadically and still remain overweight. Even if the parent doesn't try to impose these extreme behaviors on a child, the child gets the message that fat is bad.

Sometimes the messages children get are more directly aimed at them. An unthinking adult tells a child she eats too much or looks like she's gained weight. Or a classmate taunts a chubby child with names like "fatso" and "tubby." These kinds of comments can sensitize a child to her weight and cause her to become afraid of being fat. It may be that she didn't think about her weight until someone else made her feel there was something wrong with her because of it. It's important for parents to know how to talk to their children about these issues, so we'll help you with some strategies later in the book.

Fear of fat is often translated into an aversion to fat in food. Let's face it, in our society, fat is seen as the enemy, whereas low fat is touted as our savior. It's ironic that one word has come to describe a person's whole diet: It's low-fat this and low-fat that. Now don't get us wrong, eating a low fat-diet is healthy for both adults and children over two. The problem is when attitudes about eating focus on low fat to the exclusion of nutrition. Every day, in the name of good health and weight control, people eat low-fat diets (under 30 percent of calories from fat) that don't come close to providing proper nutrition.

What Does a Bad Diet Look Like?

Our bodies, young and old, need six essential nutrients: protein, fat, carbohydrates, vitamins, minerals, and water. We have to have them all in the proper amounts in order to live, and in the case of children, in order to grow. While adults can go on short-term, nutrient-restricted diets, usually without long-term harmful effects, similar diets imposed on children can be devastating.

Bad diets have different names and wear many different disguises. But, underneath, they all share one or more of these features:

1. *A bad diet is too strict.* A diet that doesn't allow a person to eat the kinds of normal food that other family members eat is too strict. One that forbids desserts or snacks also falls into this category. A diet that is too strict is impossible to stick with.

2. *A bad diet restricts calories too much.* A diet that is too low in calories is usually also too low in some of the essential nutrients we mentioned above. If a growing child is not allowed to eat enough of a variety of foods, there is no way he can get sufficient nutrients necessary for optimal growth. In addition, severe calorie restriction will cause a body to lose weight, but it will lose more muscle than fat. Not only is this loss unhealthy, but reducing muscle (lean body tissue) tends to slow metabolism and make a weight problem even more difficult to solve.

3. *A bad diet contains too little protein.* Some bad diets restrict calories and rely too much on fruits, cereals, and grains while neglecting protein and other vital nutrients. In fact, protein is the nutrient that suffers most often when calories are restricted. When a child's diet is too low in calories, the protein that is eaten is burned to meet the energy requirements of daily living, rather than used for growth. Children need protein to build all body tissue, including bone and muscle. It is also essential for proper maintenance of the body's immune system.

4. *A bad diet skips meals.* Not only should children eat three meals a day, they also need a couple of snacks in between. Going too long between meals or skipping breakfast is a setup for overeating later in the day.

5. *A bad diet includes the consumption of pills or herbal preparations that are purported to aid weight loss.* Many of these preparations, even those labeled "organic" or "herbal," contain ingredients that can be harmful to children and adults.

6. *A bad diet results in too-rapid weight loss.* You can tell if a diet is too strict if it causes rapid weight loss. Weight loss for adults should generally not progress faster than two pounds a week. Children, if they lose weight at all, should do so at a much slower pace.

7. *A bad diet lasts for a specific period of time.* Most diets share this

feature—a short-term mentality. For every diet that someone goes on, they also eventually go off it. The best way to achieve weight control is to change how you eat in a way that will last for the rest of your life. Temporary fixes don't work for anyone, adults or children.

8. *A bad diet doesn't include exercise.* The surest way to make a weight problem worse is to restrict calories and limit exercise. These two actions, separately, but especially together, act to slow a person's metabolism, making it even harder to lose weight.

Don't Restrict Kids the Wrong Way

A bad diet featuring the components we outlined above is not healthy for an adult, although many adults do punish themselves with such regimens. Children should never be subjected to such a diet. Why? Because strict diets, with calorie restrictions that result in poor nutrition, can stunt a child's growth and, in some cases, this stunting can be irreversible.

Even if your attempts to restrict your child's food are not severe enough to slow his growth, over-controlling your child's eating could backfire in other ways. It could create a child who is worried all the time that he's going to go hungry. When food is restricted, children tend to overeat whenever they get a chance. A child who is hungry will do whatever it takes to get food—sneak it, beg for it, scrounge it—and he may eat more than if you didn't try to control his food volume in the first place. At the other extreme, there is evidence that strict dieting, with the deprivation it produces, may promote eating disorders in children.

We know you don't want to take any chances with your child. That's why we have to approach your child's weight control in a cautious, conservative, healthy way. We will show you how to incorporate changes gradually, so you don't compromise your child's good nutrition or optimal growth.

If you saw yourself in some of the examples we've given, and think you may be restricting your child's eating too much, don't panic. Most likely, you haven't done anything that has caused permanent damage. Just be sure you stop now, until you've learned enough from this book to help your child lose weight the healthy way.

It's Okay for Your Child to Lose Fat

Some overweight children can lose a few pounds in a healthy way. All chubby children, even if they don't need to lose weight, can afford to get rid of some fat while gaining some muscle. Our balanced approach to weight control, which includes a modest reduction in calories, adequate protein, less fat and sugar, and more exercise, can do just that.

This is how it works. When you provide good nutrition (including adequate protein, vitamins, and minerals) for healthy growth and reduce calories modestly, an overweight child will get the extra energy she needs from her excess body fat. One way to make sure that you are not reducing calories too much is to be sure that weight loss occurs slowly. This is important because slow weight loss ensures that growth is not being compromised. It also demonstrates that the changes in eating and exercise are not so extreme or unpleasant that a child will be unable or unwilling to make them a part of her life.

Positive changes in food and fitness should be your goal—not changes on the bathroom scale. If you focus on good eating and enough physical activity, the scale will take care of itself. Also, if your child gains muscle and loses fat, he will look thinner and be more fit, but he won't necessarily weigh less. That's because muscle weighs more than fat but takes up less space.

Learn a Lesson With Your Child

As we've said before, we're going to teach you how to make changes in the lifestyle patterns of your family. The reason for this focus is that every research study on the subject demonstrates that weight control programs where the parents make the same kinds of changes as the overweight child result in the greatest long-term success. Also, such programs do not negatively affect the growth of the children.

If you and your spouse are perennial dieters, here's an opportunity to give up dieting for good. It is also an opportunity to get yourself into a healthier eating pattern. By doing so, you can serve as a positive role model for your child. Children really respond to "do as I do, not just as I say."

What if Your Child Has Put Herself on a "Diet"?

In a study of fourth-grade children, 60 percent of girls and 38 percent of boys wanted to be thinner. Eighty percent of all the children reported that they sometimes or very often kept themselves from eating food they thought might make them fat, while 41 percent said they had gone on a diet to lose weight. Another study of teenagers revealed that nearly half of the high school senior boys and almost three-quarters of the senior girls had dieted and lost five pounds or more.

If your child has put herself on a diet, it's likely to be overly restricted in calories and lacking in proper nutrition. What does a teenager's "diet" look like? Teenage girls, in particular, tend to cut down on total calories, and often they do it by eating only the food they like best. She might skip breakfast, eat a light lunch of chips and a soda, and have a salad for dinner. But after three days she's starving, so she'll chow down on pizza with her friends.

The danger is that some children have the ability to endure the hunger, in their quest to be thinner. This kind of restricted energy intake among pre-adolescents not only can retard growth and sexual development, it also can have harmful effects on learning, the child's ability to concentrate, and school performance.

If your child is trying to lose weight because she's overweight or because she fears she's going to get fat, you can help. One strategy is to share this book with her and tell her that you'll help her control her weight in a healthy way. You'll need to convince her that you only want to be sure she stays healthy—that it's not about her weight. If you can secure her trust, you can help her make appropriate changes that will allow her to lose weight and feel better about herself.

If she is resistant to your suggestions of prudent weight control, you may want to show her the following sentence. If a teenager restricts her calories and nutrition, she may be compromising the *last chance* she has to grow taller. This may be the only thing that will convince her not to go on a strict diet. Adults often joke, "I wouldn't be overweight if only I were a couple of inches taller." Well, in the case of teenagers, they may indeed have the ability to grow a couple of more inches—and not be overweight.

9

The Leapfrog Course
of Height and Weight

CHILDREN GROW continuously, but they don't grow in equal increments. One year a child may sprout up three inches and grow only one inch the next; he may gain four pounds one year and two pounds the next. You might think that in a year when a child grows three inches, he also would gain more weight than in a year when he only grows one inch. This sounds logical, but it isn't necessarily the way it works.

Sometimes the height comes before weight gain. But sometimes the weight gain takes place before the inches are added. It may be normal for an individual child to gain weight before his height, so that his weight will normalize by the time he's fully grown. However, the other scenario for a weight gain that occurs before an increase in height may be related to an excessive intake of calories.

Because you don't know which course *your* child will follow, it's prudent to focus on controlling overweight while ensuring that normal growth takes place in *either* case.

With a thin child, the calories to support growth have to come from food, while a pudgier youngster can use the extra calories she has stored in the form of fat to help fuel her growth. Luckily the human body doesn't care where the calories come from, as long it gets enough of them. Therefore, the goal for your overweight child is to obtain adequate nutrition, including protein, vitamins, and minerals, while using up some of the excess fat for the energy to grow.

And growing takes a lot of energy. On average, boys grow most from ages twelve through sixteen. During that time they have a good chance of getting twelve inches taller and fifty to sixty pounds heavier. They achieve most of their height by the time they are eighteen to twenty years old and they continue to put on weight from added muscle for about two years after that.

Girls grow fastest from ages ten through fourteen, during which time the average girl gets ten inches taller and gains forty to fifty pounds. After that time, they grow slowly in height and put on a bit more weight, primarily in the form of fat.

To illustrate how chubby children can grow out of their extra weight, here are the stories of three children. The first two demonstrate how moderate changes in diet and exercise can produce successful results. The third is an example of how an extreme approach can result in dire consequences.

Philip

When Philip was five years old, he was at the 85th percentile, meaning he was moderately overweight. Unfortunately, Philip's parents had no way of predicting Philip's future. They didn't know whether (1) he was going to grow an inch in the next six months, while remaining the same weight, and end up at the 50th percentile for BMI; (2) he was going to stay the same for the next six months; or (3) he was going to keep his same height, but continue to gain weight, resulting in his being at the 95th percentile for BMI— seriously overweight. Since they could not predict the future, they decided to take prudent steps to ensure both optimal growth and weight control.

A closer look at Philip reveals three older siblings (two brothers and a sister) and a family life where the mother does the cooking. None of Philip's siblings were chubby, so Mom had never paid attention to the types of snacks and foods available to any of the kids. Snacks consisted of various types of chips, nuts, and other high-fat foods, as well as plenty of sweets. The whole family was used to eating meals together and grabbing snacks whenever they wanted. Philip, being the littlest child, had to gobble up his food quickly in order to get seconds of his favorite foods, before his big brothers got what was left in the dish. Philip was not that overweight at five, but he certainly was developing habits that could easily have made him seriously overweight when he grew up. So here are some things his parents started to do to help keep that from happening.

As you will see, the whole family was involved in the process, which may, at first, seem as though the whole family had to "sacrifice" for little Philip. But we challenge you to think of it in terms of the whole family "benefiting." After all, it's healthier for everyone, whatever weight, to eat better.

First, they gradually cut down on how many bags of cookies and potato chips they brought into the house and how often. They found healthier alternatives, such as pretzels and popcorn, which were equally acceptable to the kids' tastebuds, but lower in fat and higher in nutrition. Mom prepared lots of extra vegetables and grains, which are healthy and low-calorie, in order to ensure plenty of food for whoever needed second helpings. But at the same time she fixed just enough of the higher-fat foods for everyone to have only one serving, bypassing the temptation for seconds. A child who was still hungry could always have an extra slice of bread or piece of fruit.

These moderate changes resulted in Philip's growing out of his extra weight by the time he had his checkup at six years old.

Ruth

At sixteen years old, Ruth is just right—at 5 feet 4 inches and 125 pounds. But she hasn't always been at this healthy weight for her height. As a child, she was small and petite, and her parents assumed she would be this way for her whole life. All the girls in the class were bigger than Ruth until she was eleven years old, when she started to eat, gain weight, and grow inches at a very rapid rate.

At twelve, she started to get chubby and worry about her weight. So her mother helped her by providing the right food environment at home. Since Ruth had always been able to satisfy her desire for sweets, cutting back on cookies, ice cream, and candy was especially difficult. To make matters worse, Ruth's mother had an incurable sweet tooth and kept it well supplied. At any given moment there were hordes of candy bars in the house and everyone knew where to find them. In time, Mom managed to rid the house of candy and other high-fat sweets, knowing that she could indulge herself when she was out of the house. The next step was to convert the remaining high-fat sweets to lower-fat alternatives. For example, ice cream became frozen yogurt; Oreos became fat-free chocolate chip cookies; and cake was traded for lower-fat versions.

The other dilemma for Ruth was that she wanted to slim down but not call attention to herself in social situations by eating differently than her friends. She and her friends traded houses for their Saturday night sleepovers. The problem was that all of the kids offered the usual chips, cookies, and sodas, but no other choices. So gradually she started bringing extra snacks for herself and her friends—things like grapes, pretzels, popcorn, and some of her low-fat cookies. Although she felt awkward at first, controlling her weight was so important to her that she overcame her fear of being different.

However, when they decided to go out for pizza, Ruth couldn't resist eating along with her friends. If she knew in advance, she ate a low-fat snack at home before she met her friends. That way, she was able to limit herself to one piece of pizza. When it was a spur-of-the-moment pizza, she figured out that by ordering a salad, she would be able to eat less pizza.

When they started seventh grade, Ruth and her friends tried out for the volleyball team. Playing on the team became a big part of her social life and also introduced her to the positive effects of exercise. Her father, knowing that exercise was the other half of weight control, volunteered to pick up the girls after practice.

With the changes in her food and exercise habits, by the age of thirteen, when she started her menstrual period, she was only a little chubby. She had gotten taller and even had more inches to grow. Now, at sixteen, she is finished growing and has learned the habits that will help keep her at a healthy weight for her whole life.

Elizabeth

Elizabeth's mother has always paid attention to her own weight and food choices. Elizabeth has heard her mother and father comment negatively about "fat people" all her life. When Elizabeth was a little girl, at birthday parties, her mother used to grab cake out of her hands saying, "You don't need this—you're too fat!" At restaurants, Elizabeth used to open packets of sugar and eat them when her parents weren't looking. At a very young age, food became a loaded issue for her.

Elizabeth's mother was tall and thin, but her father was stockier. It frustrated her mother that Elizabeth was chubby like her father, especially since her older sister was thin like her mother. Her mother nagged her about her weight and her eating, perhaps more often than she realized. Consequently, when Elizabeth turned twelve, like the rest of her friends, she started worrying about her looks. Six months later, when she was 5 feet 2 inches and had reached 130 pounds, she decided to go on a diet. First, her parents were pleased and encouraged her efforts to exercise more and eat less.

However, as time went on, she would refuse the family food at dinner, choosing instead to eat just a plate of vegetables. Her lunches dwindled to a piece of fruit and a diet soda. Elizabeth, at this point, started rapidly losing large amounts of weight. Since it had been so hard for her to lose weight earlier in her life, she was quite pleased with her progress and delighted with how she looked. It amazed everyone that she could refuse her favorite foods all of the time. But, eventually, her parents became worried, because it seemed to them that Elizabeth was becoming obsessed with getting thinner and thinner.

Although she started her period two months before her thirteenth birthday, shortly thereafter she had gotten down to 105 pounds and stopped menstruating. Studies clearly show that when a young girl stops menstruating, she starts losing calcium from her bones and compromises her critical adolescent growth spurt. Losing twenty-five pounds in six months may be commendable for an adult, but it is dangerous for a growing teenager.

At thirteen and a half, one year after she started dieting, she was still 5 feet 2 inches, but weighed only 88 pounds. Although her parents had taken her to see her doctor and a nutritionist, Elizabeth resisted their advice to gain weight. She was so focused on her looks that she didn't want to acknowledge the fact that her poor diet and extreme weight loss were damaging her health and stunting her growth. It was at this time that she was referred for professional counseling and was diagnosed with the eating disorder anorexia nervosa.

What About Your Child?

We told you these stories to give you hope about your child's future growth and, at the same time, to alert you to the dangers of extreme dieting. But, remember, your child is not Ruth, Philip, Elizabeth, or any other youngster. He is a unique individual with his own personality, behaviors, food preferences, exercise habits, and sensitivities. So although the basic concepts of weight control are the same for all children, the ways you apply them to help *your* child have to be tailored to his needs and issues. And in order to be successful, they will have to be compatible with the lifestyle of your family.

You will need to focus some energy on this task to make it work. As we get into the "how-to's," we'll refer you back to the assessments you did in chapters 4, 5, and 7. In the next part, "Focus on Food," we'll ask you to analyze your child's Food Records and Eating Behavior Survey. Your child's Activity Assessment as well as the Family Favorites Chart will be important tools when we get to part IV, "Focus on Fitness." And, from time to time, throughout the rest of the book, we will ask you to consider Your Family Portrait to help pinpoint the strategies that are likely to be most effective for you and your child.

We know this won't be easy. But we'll help you every step of the way by offering strategies for healthy weight control. Some solutions will be right for your child; others may not be. Sometimes you'll just have to try an idea to see if it works. Remember, don't force the changes or try to make too many at one time. And, above all, be sure that you are supporting and nurturing your child throughout the entire process.

PART III

Focus on Food

10

Food Roles, Responsibilities, and Rights

"There is no love sincerer than the love of food."

—GEORGE BERNARD SHAW,
Man and Superman, Act I

WHILE MR. SHAW may have exaggerated a bit, there is no denying that food gratifies us under adverse conditions; it makes us feel happy; we celebrate with food; and we can't live without it. As we begin our focus on food, we want to share with you our philosophy about the rights of children, the responsibilities of parents, and the roles both can play in relation to food.

In the broadest sense, it is a parent's responsibility to manage the "food environment," to make sure that nutritious food is available to the child on a reliable basis and that it is presented in a positive manner. It then becomes the child's right to contribute to determining how much, if any, he is going to eat. While the fulfillment of these responsibilities and rights will vary somewhat depending upon the child, the situation, and the family, they are the foundation for helping any child, chubby or not, grow up healthy.

Children's Bill of Rights

When it comes to eating, children have four basic rights that should be respected and supported by their parents. In supporting these rights, it is also the responsibility of parents to be sure that they are applied in a reasonable and realistic manner.

1. *Children have the right not to go hungry or endure deprivation.* This doesn't mean that a child can't get hungry or be hungry at times

79

during the day. In fact, it's desirable for a child to be hungry when she sits down to eat a meal or a snack. What is *not* acceptable is for a child to be deprived of food in the name of weight control or as a form of punishment for misbehavior. A child who is forced to go hungry may become fearful that she won't get enough to eat. If she is frequently subjected to hunger, she might become overly concerned about food, sneak food, and overeat when food is available. It's not hard to see how such behavior could contribute to unhealthy weight gain.

2. *Children have the right to choose among the foods available.* It is a parent's responsibility to provide nutritious food that is suitable for the child and to present it in a pleasing way. It is the child's right to choose the ones that he wants to eat. While it's appropriate to ask your child to try new foods, no child should be forced to eat something he finds distasteful.

The key is to offer your children a variety of foods. We're not talking about being a short-order cook, but rather providing a variety of options at each meal. That way, if your child doesn't like the sweet potatoes you served for dinner, he can eat a slice of bread; if he hates the peas, he can have extra salad. Or when you pack your child's lunch box, ask if she would prefer a turkey, tuna, or cheese sandwich and if she'd rather have grapes, an apple, or a banana. There's nothing that says you have to offer a multiple choice of candy, cookies, and cake.

3. *Children have the right to eat as much or as little as they need.* This notion may fly in the face of what you believe about a child's ability to sense when he's hungry or gauge when he's full. We acknowledge that children aren't *always* reliable judges of what's best for them: They may not be able to tell when they need to take a bath, go to sleep, or do their homework. But when it comes to knowing when their body hurts or when they are hungry, they are no less accurate than adults are.

We know that this may go against your gut feeling that, as a parent, you will have to restrict the amount of food your child eats in order to help him with his weight. But we ask you to look at the evidence and reconsider your position. Research studies have demonstrated that children whose food intake was restricted were more likely to be overweight than children who were not limited in the amount of food they were allowed to eat. Some of the overweight children in the studies were unable to regulate their own food intake because their parents had always done it for them.

The reason for this may be that over-controlling a child's eating can eventually override the internal cues that signal hunger and satiety. If this has already happened to your child, she may not be able to accurately tell when she's hungry or satisfied. As a result, when you first give her the right to control her own food volume, she may overeat. But work with her and see if she can moderate the volume of food she eats, especially when she trusts that she won't have to go hungry.

One way to help your child exercise his right to control how much he eats is to allow him to serve his own plate. Although this might be a bit messy with a young child whose coordination isn't very well developed, you can help steady the spoon until he gets more proficient.

Another option is to serve modest portions of the selections your child says she wants and tell her that she can have second helpings if she's still hungry. But you may have to step in if she wants thirds. In chapter 16, we'll offer you strategies for helping your child with volume and portion size.

4. *Children have the right to enjoy their favorite foods.* This doesn't mean that a child can have chocolate chip cookies for breakfast, lunch, and dinner, or that he has to have potato chips in his lunch box every day. What it means is that chocolate chip cookies, potato chips, and all the other things your child loves to eat shouldn't be banished from his life. In order to grow up with healthy eating habits, children have to learn how to eat cookies, as well as carrots. You can help teach your child that the key to enjoying those favorite foods that are high in calories or low in nutrition is moderation—in both amount and frequency.

Parents' Responsibilities

As you read about the responsibilities you have with respect to food, don't panic. We don't expect you to become Ozzie and Harriet. Our guess is that you will recognize a number of roles that you are already performing well. What you need to consider are the actions you may not be taking sufficient responsibility for, and how this may be affecting your child's eating.

Throughout the book, whenever we suggest that you consider modifying an attitude or behavior, we want you to make incremental changes. Don't do anything drastic, such as switching abruptly from whole milk to fat-free or dumping all the chips down the disposal.

In fact, even if you could change everything all at once, it wouldn't be as effective as making a series of small adjustments. The reason is that you can better gauge the success of one change at a time and modify your strategy as you go along. If one suggestion doesn't work, try another until you find the solution that's best for your child and the entire family.

We've said it before, but it bears repeating: It is critical that your chubby child not be singled out for "special treatment." Any changes you make and any new rules or policies you institute must be applied as equally as possible to all members of the family.

In your role as "change agent," you should try to keep everyone reasonably happy—your child, your spouse, your other children, and yourself. Try to prevent yourself from becoming a drill sergeant ordering changes left and right. Instead, imagine that you're a diplomat, working behind the scenes to make things happen without ruffling any feathers. By making subtle changes, it will not only be easier on you, but you'll be able to make a lot of positive strides without anyone noticing.

However, sooner or later someone in the family is going to ask you a pointed question like, "Why is there only frozen yogurt in the freezer?" You need to be prepared with a better answer than, "It was on sale." And whatever you do, don't make your overweight child the scapegoat. After all, you're trying to help the whole family be healthier. Maybe that should be your response.

As we said, parents are in charge of managing the "food environment" in which their children live. In this role, you have a variety of responsibilities.

1. *Learn about good nutrition.* This may sound obvious, but in order to provide good nutrition for your child's growth and health, you need to know what kinds of foods make up a well-balanced diet. While you don't need to analyze the folic acid and zinc content of each item you put in your shopping cart, you should learn how to

use the concept of the Food Pyramid to provide proper nutrition for your child's development. We will be discussing this in detail in chapter 12, when we'll "Climb the Food Pyramid" together.

2. *You have the responsibility for grocery shopping.* Since having nutritious food in the house is a parent's responsibility, you'll need to play the lead role in grocery shopping. If both spouses buy food, be sure you are in agreement about these general shopping objectives; we will get into the specifics in later chapters.

- Plan in advance and make a shopping list to control impulse buying.
- Read labels. Learn what they can tell you about nutrition, calories, and fat, and how they also can be misleading.
- Buy a variety of foods. Children learn to eat what is available to them, and eating a greater variety of foods helps contribute to good nutrition.
- Purchase more low-fat foods, but don't buy food your child doesn't like just because it's low-fat or fat-free.
- Buy fewer high-fat, high-sugar items, and buy them less often. The fewer temptations in the house, the better. However, cutting out all high-calorie foods will just make your child, and the rest of the family, want them more.
- Keep ahead of your kitchen inventory so you don't run out of healthy options and then have to stop for pizza or Chinese food for the third night in a row.
- Take your children with you to the supermarket from time to time. Not only will it help them learn about new foods that are healthier for them, *you* will learn more about the foods they like. Also, when children are involved in choosing the food, they tend to be happier about eating it.

3. *Create a food environment that doesn't trigger unnecessary eating.* The issue here is that it's human nature to want to eat something that looks appetizing. Having sweets or other high-fat, high-calorie foods out in plain view is a setup for eating them, even when we're not hungry. For many children, as well as adults, the sight of food stimulates an otherwise dormant appetite. You can help your chubby child by storing away such tempting goodies. You know the old saying: Out of sight, out of mind.

Fortunately, you can make food availability work in a positive way. For example, by keeping low-fat, high-fiber foods readily available and in plain view, you will ensure that your children won't feel that there's nothing in the house to eat. And you can increase the odds that they will grab an apple for a snack if it's washed and displayed prominently in a bowl on the kitchen table. This is especially true if the cookies are in a tin, on a hard-to-reach top shelf, above the stove.

4. *Prepare food wisely.* You don't have to be a gourmet chef, unless you want to be. Just try to prepare healthful foods that suit the tastes of your family.

One slimming strategy is to gradually cut down on the fat you use in cooking. For example, if a recipe calls for three tablespoons of oil, try making it with two tablespoons next time. If that works okay, try the recipe with one tablespoon. You don't have to cut the fat out completely, just get it as low as possible without sacrificing taste.

Another important responsibility of the cook is to refrain from serving huge amounts of food that make seconds and thirds more enticing. If you want to cook extra for a second meal, wrap one half and put it immediately in the refrigerator or freezer before you serve the other half to your family.

Children can play a role in preparing food. Depending upon his age, a child can push the buttons on the microwave, toss the salad, or cut up vegetables. He is more likely to eat, or at least try, foods that he helped prepare.

5. *Emphasize mealtimes and provide appropriate snacks.* One research study looking for differences in children's diets found a significant factor that distinguished thin youngsters from overweight children: The thinner children had more structure in their meals and snacks.

Try to schedule meals so that everyone in the family knows when they can expect to eat, especially when dinner will be on the table. Meals don't have to be at the same time each day, as long as your children know when they are going to be served. Don't let children skip meals, or they will be that much hungrier when the next opportunity to eat comes around, creating another setup for *over*eating.

Snacks are especially important for children, whose small stomachs and high energy needs make it impossible to go for a long time without eating. By a snack, we don't mean a handful of chips or a can of soda. A snack should be nourishing, healthy, large enough to ease the child's hunger, and satisfying enough to last until the next planned meal. We'll give you a lot more ideas and information about snacks as we continue to focus on food.

6. *Make mealtimes pleasant.* Mealtimes, especially dinner, can be pleasant functions or dreaded experiences for your child. If the dinner table tends to be the site of arguments or lectures, make a decision with your spouse to avoid talking about unpleasant subjects at mealtime. If your child is having trouble in school, discuss her grades and homework after dinner. And you may have to make a special effort not to pick at her about what she's eating.

We know that everyone has busy schedules these days, but try to have dinner together as a family whenever possible, at least once a week. And it doesn't count if everyone's watching television. The idea is to enjoy one another's company and share pleasant conversations along with the food.

And try to make family meals last more than fifteen minutes. Not only is this more conducive to conversation, but, by eating slowly, your child may discover that he is satisfied and can stop before he's overeaten. Some studies indicate that overweight children tend to eat faster than thinner children.

7. *Role-model good food behaviors.* Most food behaviors are learned, not inborn; and parents are the most influential teachers of both good and bad food habits. Here are a few good habits to try to model for your children:

- Take moderate portions of foods, rather than overloading your plate.
- Don't skip meals.
- Eat slowly, enjoying your food—do not gobble it.
- Try new foods—be open to experimenting.
- Eat a piece of fruit for dessert sometimes, instead of a sweet.
- Don't drink soda at a meal if you expect your child to drink milk or water.

8. *Do not use food to reward or punish.* Discipline is a part of parenting, but it's very important not to use food in connection with punishment. As we said in the Children's Bill of Rights, withholding

food can create anxiety, causing your child to worry that he will not get enough to eat or that he will have to endure hunger.

Rewarding with food can be just as harmful for a child, especially one with a weight problem. When a child is repeatedly rewarded with sweets or some other high-sugar or high-fat food, she will come to believe that these foods are better than other, more healthful foods. We read with dismay the suggestion in our local newspaper that M&Ms be used to reward a child for making progress with potty training.

It's a double whammy when parents reward a child with dessert for cleaning his plate. It gives the message that eating a larger volume of food is desirable and that dessert is better than the rest of dinner. These kinds of "fat habits" are difficult to change and may persist throughout a child's lifetime.

9. *Be flexible and understanding.* It's up to you to be flexible and understanding while you and your family are trying to change your food dynamics. No one is perfect: We all have days when our best-laid plans fall apart. When these things happen, give yourself a break, give your child a hug, and start fresh.

Making changes takes sincere effort. But remember: It's easier to make gradual changes than abrupt ones; it's smarter to make one change at a time than to make ten; and it's more effective over time to ease into new, moderate habits than it is to force practices that are too extreme to live with.

11

There's No Such Thing as Good Foods or Bad Foods

"BE A GOOD GIRL, eat your spinach." "No, you can't have a piece of candy, it's bad for you." These kinds of parental proclamations are made every day, but they're not really accurate. Eating spinach doesn't make a girl good, any more than eating cake makes her bad. And candy isn't really bad for you, unless you overdo it. Food is neither good nor bad, it's just food. And people, regardless of their age, are neither good nor bad because of what they eat.

This isn't to say that all food is equal, but we'll get to that a little later. First we want to discuss why it's important to teach your child about food without calling some foods "good" and others "bad."

Almost as soon as they can speak, children are able to label food as yummy or yucky. It's a simple determination—yummy tastes good and yucky tastes bad.

Unfortunately, many adults have come to perceive some food that tastes good as being bad for them, and they pass this idea on to their children. This erroneous notion probably stems from the "eat this, but don't eat that" approach to weight loss that is imposed by most diets. Not surprisingly, many of our favorite foods—from hamburgers and French fries, to cake and ice cream—are on the "don't eat" list and have to be given up for the duration of the diet. As a way of coping with this prohibition, dieters may convince themselves that the reason they can't eat these foods is that they are fattening, therefore bad. Even when they go off the diet, they may still think of all high-fat, high-calorie foods as bad or bad for them.

But our approach to helping your chubby child is not a diet, remember? Rather, our program involves living *with* food, not living without it. So you have to help your child learn how to eat French fries and ice cream as well as fruits and vegetables.

That's because food is an integral part of life: It satisfies real needs in people of all ages, not only physical nourishment, but sensory enjoyment and emotional comfort as well. If food only had to provide sustenance for our bodies, it could be packaged in tablets that we would swallow with a glass of water. But who would want to give up the enjoyment of food? Nobody. Savoring the taste of food is one of the pleasures of being alive. We even use the term "comfort food" to describe those most delicious, homey foods we remember from our childhood—the foods that make us feel good, that provide us with solace and even ease our stress. It wouldn't be fair to deprive our children of *their* favorite foods.

All Foods Are Not Created Equal

Although specific foods are neither bad nor good, foods do vary in a wide variety of other ways. Some foods taste better than others; some have more vitamins; some have more protein or carbohydrate; some have more fiber or calcium; some have more calories and some have more fat. That's why it's important for children to eat a variety of foods. It is the only way they can get enough of all the nutrients they need to grow.

But eating a wide variety of foods doesn't guarantee that your child won't be eating too many calories or too much fat.

Where's the Fat?

When we talk about fat in food, we're referring to the percent of total calories in the food that are derived from fat. Most health organizations recommend that no more than 30 percent of the calories a person consumes come from fat. This recommendation also applies to children over two years of age.

In later chapters, we will talk a lot about fat, from how to figure percent fat to low-fat substitutions for traditionally high-fat foods. But for now, we want to give you the big picture of fat so you can see

The Big Picture of Fat

Butter, all oils, margarine, mayonnaise (except for reduced-fat products)	100%
Bacon, sausage, high-fat lunch meats, hot dogs, avocado	80–95%
Corn chips, potato chips, tortilla chips, nuts, coconut, trail mix, peanut butter, and other nut butters	65–95%
High-fat cheeses: American, bleu, Brie, cheddar, cream cheese, Monterey Jack, Parmesan, Roquefort, Swiss	65–90%
Red meats: beef, lamb, pork (most cuts); whole eggs	50–70%
Cake, cookies, crackers, chocolate candy, desserts, ice cream, pastries	50–70%
Reduced-fat cheeses (less than 6 grams of fat per ounce), whole milk	50–55%
Dark meat chicken or turkey with skin	45–50%
Dark meat chicken or turkey without skin, white meat chicken or turkey with skin, 2% milk	35–45%
Higher-fat fish: carp, catfish, salmon, sturgeon, swordfish, tuna in oil	30–40%
Top round steak (London broil), eye of the round roast	25%
Light meat chicken or turkey without skin	20%
Lower-fat dairy products: 1% milk, low-fat cottage cheese, low-fat yogurt, low-fat frozen yogurt	10–20%
Lower-fat fish: all shellfish, cod, halibut, mahi-mahi, orange roughy, sea bass, snapper, sole, trout, tuna in water	6–20%
Starches: breads, rolls, cereals, pasta, rice, low-fat crackers, baked tortilla chips, baked potato chips, pretzels	5–15%
Beans, lentils	5%
Fat-free dairy products: fat-free milk, fat-free yogurt, fat-free frozen yogurt, fat-free ice cream, fat-free cottage cheese; egg whites	0–6%
Vegetables (including potatoes)	none
Fruits (even bananas)	none

where the food your family eats fits into this picture. You'll discover that some of the foods contain 0 percent fat and some are 100 percent fat, while most fall somewhere in between.

You'll notice that we didn't draw a line at 30 percent and label those above the line as bad and those below as good. That's because, although 30 percent of calories from fat is the *overall* goal, it's appropriate to eat food at every percentage—even those that are 100 percent fat.

Are you surprised that we don't even consider pure fat to be bad? The reason is that, from a nutritional standpoint, our bodies require a certain amount of fat. Fat is an essential nutrient, needed to maintain life. If we labeled pure fat as "bad," it would mean that you could never use oil in cooking and that your child could never put margarine on a slice of toast. And that just isn't realistic for normal eating or necessary for weight loss.

Have we made our point? Okay, now we can make the *real* point, which is: *Just because foods that are high in fat are not "bad" doesn't mean it's okay for your child to eat them as often or as much as he may want.* Here's where it gets tricky. You have to help your child learn how to eat higher-fat foods in smaller amounts and to eat them less often than lower-fat foods. For example, if she loves margarine on her toast, she can use a smaller amount. Or, as a trade-off, maybe she can try low-fat sour cream on her baked potato instead of more margarine.

And since moderation is the goal, it's important to realize that, just like adults, children tend to crave foods they think they cannot have and may be tempted to overeat them when they get the chance. If you've ever gone on a "diet," you know that the forbidden foods are the ones you want the most. Even though a bowl of fresh, ripe strawberries is delicious, it doesn't seem nearly as enticing as the "forbidden" bowl of strawberry ice cream.

Labeling food that you want your child to eat more often as "good" and ones you want her to eat less often as "bad" can backfire in a variety of ways. One research study found that when children were praised by a parent for trying a new food, they were *less* likely to try it the next time it was offered than were children whose parent made no comment.

All kinds of thoughts can go through a child's mind. When young-sters hear their parents refer to some foods as good and others as bad, they may translate these ideas into such thoughts as "I'm good when I eat some foods, but I'm bad when I eat others." Or "When I want to be bad, I'll eat candy and soda; when I want to be good, I'll eat vegetables and drink milk." Or even "I feel bad, so it doesn't matter if I eat a lot of cookies, because I'm already bad." Children can even use eating so-called bad food as their way of rebelling against their parents.

So how are you going to talk about food if you want to keep from labeling it good or bad? First of all, try not to substitute other judgmental words, such as "low-calorie" for good, or "fattening" or "junk" for bad. Instead, think of food in terms of what's in it and how it should be eaten. No food is fattening by itself—it's only fattening if you eat too much of it or eat it too often.

The objective is to eat high-fat, high-calorie, and low-nutrition foods less often and in smaller quantities. Low-calorie, low-fat, high-nutrition foods should be chosen more often and in relatively greater amounts. When you put these objectives into action, it becomes a kind of balancing act.

Balancing Acts

There are a number of different ways to balance food. We're going to talk about the kinds of balancing acts that can have the most significant impact on your child's weight and happiness. Balance is about allow-ing your child to eat enough of her favorite foods to be happy, but eating less of the high-fat/high-calorie ones in order to lose weight the healthy way. If you want to share some of the information in this book with your child, these balance points may be a good place to start.

Balance Point 1: Balance on a daily and on a weekly basis. What your child eats at a single meal matters less than what he eats in the course of a day. And what he eats in a single day matters less than what he eats in the course of a week. This applies to calories, fat, and other nutrients.

Balance Point 2: Balance high fat with low fat. The goal is to end up with your child consuming no more than 30 percent of his calorie intake from fat over the course of the week. But, we don't expect you to walk around with a calculator figuring fat. As you learn more about which foods are lower in fat and which are higher, you'll get used to buying more foods that are lower in fat. If you do this gradually, the total fat your child eats will slowly decrease.

Balance Point 3: Balance special occasions with "regular" days of the year. Work on balance on routine days, not on holidays or at family celebrations that have special foods attached to them. It is neither fair nor necessary for your child to forgo Aunt Hilda's pumpkin pie on Thanksgiving or to pass up the hot dogs and potato salad at the Fourth of July picnic. But you have to be realistic. There might be only three to four special occasion days each month: New Year's Day, Valentine's Day, Easter, Memorial Day, Independence Day, Labor Day, Halloween, Thanksgiving, the day after Thanksgiving, Christmas Eve, Christmas, New Year's Eve, family birthdays, friends' birthdays, and, perhaps, other special family or school celebrations.

Balance Point 4: Balance taste preferences. If your child is trying to control her weight, she may not be able to have her number one taste choice every single time. She'll need to balance high-fat foods that taste delicious with low-fat foods that she likes too. This balance point will be more difficult to implement if your youngster is not actively involved in changing her eating habits. But don't worry, we'll help you find subtle ways to substitute lower fat for higher fat that your family will not dislike or maybe not even notice.

Balance Point 5: Balance treats. Please note: Treats are not rewards. They are simply high-fat foods that your child especially enjoys. Your child needs to have treats often enough not to feel deprived, but not so often that he is gaining weight from having too many. The best approach is gradual. If he is used to having ice cream every night, substitute a popsicle or Fudgesicle every other night for a few weeks. Then try to get down to having ice cream less often, perhaps once a week.

Balance Point 6: Balance empty calories with good nutrition. While foods such as soda, juice drinks, hard candy, and all the different fat-free cookies and desserts contain no fat, they are high in sugar and do not offer much in the way of nutrition. While it's acceptable for your child to eat these kinds of foods in moderation, remember that they are displacing other foods with an equal number of calories and a lot more nutrient value. A cup of 1% milk has about the same number of calories as eight ounces of cola, but instead of sugar and water, you get protein, calcium, and vitamins A and D.

Balance Point 7: Balancing isn't easy. Sometimes it's easier to do all or nothing than it is to strike a balance somewhere in between. Parents have to teach their children to balance these food issues, just as they have to teach them to balance on a bicycle. And before you let your child pedal down the sidewalk without her training wheels, you hang on to the back of the bicycle seat for a while to be sure that she's steady. The same is true with balancing food. You need to be there to support your child's efforts. You also need to pick her up when she falls off and encourage her as you gently help her get back on the bicycle.

12

Climb the Food Pyramid

WITH SO MANY FOOD PRODUCTS THESE DAYS screaming "low-fat!" "reduced-calorie!" and "fat-free!" it's easy to focus just on calories and fat while forgetting about basic nutrition. It's not good when adults trying to lose weight fall into this trap, but with children, overlooking nutrition can seriously compromise their growth.

In order to help your child grow up healthy, you may need to brush up on your nutrition knowledge. The first lesson in our Nutrition 101 class focuses on the six categories of nutrients in food that are essential to keeping the human body functioning.

Water is the most essential of the nutrients: A person can live a lot longer without food than if deprived of water. Next come the three nutrients that provide calories: carbohydrate, fat, and protein. Also known as "macro" nutrients, these three are found in abundant quantities in our food. In a child's overall diet, approximately 55 percent of total calories should come from carbohydrates, no more than 30 percent from fats, and about 15 percent from proteins.

The final two groups of essential nutrients include an assortment of more than thirty vitamins and minerals that are found in small amounts in our food. Although vitamins and minerals provide no calories, they are essential for a variety of body processes.

The good news is that these six nutrients are found in most foods; the bad news is that they are found in widely varying amounts. This is why children should eat many different kinds of foods to get all the nutrients they need. The challenge is to choose the right foods in the proper quantities to provide for optimal growth and health, without contributing to overweight.

To help with this task, the Food and Nutrition Board of the National Academy of Sciences developed the Recommended Dietary Allowances (RDAs) for many of the nutrients. You will find these Dietary Allowances reflected on food labels that indicate what percentage of the "daily values" of various nutrients the product provides. The RDAs were created to indicate the sufficient amounts of nutrients needed to maintain health and prevent various deficiency diseases caused by a lack of certain nutrients.

The United States Department of Agriculture (USDA) and the U.S. Department of Health and Human Services created the Dietary Guidelines for Americans, general philosophies about eating that are directed toward preventing the health problems of over-nutrition, as opposed to those of under-nutrition. For example, one of the Dietary Guidelines says, "Choose a diet that is low in saturated fat and cholesterol and moderate in total fat."

The problem with both of these dietary documents is that they talk about nutrients rather than about the food in which they're found. So, in 1992, the USDA created the Food Guide Pyramid, a user-friendly, pictorial way of representing how the various official nutrition recommendations and guidelines translate into real food that people eat. The Pyramid, shown on page 96, is a useful tool to help you choose food for your family that will provide appropriate amounts of all the essential nutrients.

What Happened to the Basic Four?

Remember the Basic Four Food Groups you learned about in school? For forty years, nutrition educators used the Dairy, Meat, Fruit and Vegetable, and Grain Groups as a way of teaching Americans how to get the proper foods to guard against nutrient deficiencies. The Food Guide Pyramid was developed in part to address the more prevalent problems caused by nutrient excesses.

Although both the Basic Four and the Pyramid put foods together in groups to indicate their similar nutrient content, the Pyramid has grouped the foods differently. For example, it distinguishes between vegetables and fruits, putting them in separate groups. The reason for this is that while both contain some vitamins, minerals, and fiber, only vegetables have iron and calcium. Another difference is that the

Food Guide Pyramid

A Guide to Daily Food Choices

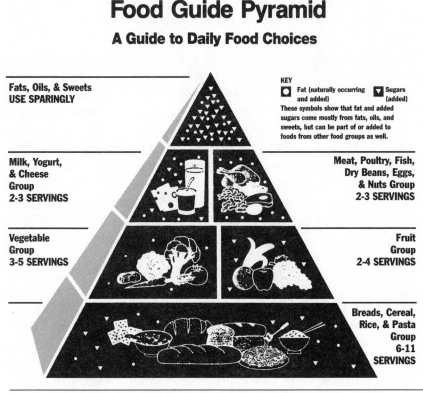

**Fats, Oils, & Sweets
USE SPARINGLY**

KEY
◻ Fat (naturally occurring and added)　▼ Sugars (added)
These symbols show that fat and added sugars come mostly from fats, oils, and sweets, but can be part of or added to foods from other food groups as well.

**Milk, Yogurt,
& Cheese
Group
2-3 SERVINGS**

**Meat, Poultry, Fish,
Dry Beans, Eggs,
& Nuts Group
2-3 SERVINGS**

**Vegetable
Group
3-5 SERVINGS**

**Fruit
Group
2-4 SERVINGS**

**Breads, Cereal,
Rice, & Pasta
Group
6-11
SERVINGS**

Source: U.S. Department of Agriculture/U.S. Department of Health and Human Services

combined recommended number of vegetables and fruits is greater on the Pyramid than with the Basic Four in order to reflect the importance of the nutrients and fiber they provide.

The servings of dairy and protein have remained basically the same, but the Pyramid recommends more grains than the Basic Four did. This recommendation supports the suggested decrease in fats, oils, and sweets, which is in keeping with medical research findings and health advice of the last two decades.

Why a Pyramid Shape?

The Food Guide Pyramid's form is integral to its function. Not only is each of its four levels a different size—getting smaller as we get closer to the top—but each has a unique significance.

Level 1, the Bread, Cereal, Rice, and Pasta Group, represents the food group from which we should eat the most servings (six to eleven) and derive the greatest percentage of calories in our total diet. This bottom level forms a secure base in terms of volume and low-fat nutrition. As we go up the Pyramid, the levels get smaller, indicating that we should eat fewer servings of the foods on the higher levels.

Level 2 contains the Vegetable Group and the Fruit Group, and you'll notice that the Vegetable Group is slightly larger than the Fruit Group. This shows that there should be more servings from the Vegetable Group (three to five) than the Fruit Group (two to four).

When we get to Level 3, with the Milk, Yogurt, and Cheese Group and the Meat, Poultry, Fish, Dry Beans, Eggs, and Nuts Group, the two boxes are of equal size, but smaller than either the Vegetables or the Fruits. It isn't that they are less important. Rather, the nutrients we need from these groups can be obtained from two to three servings a day. Also, by the time we get to Level 3, there may be more fat per serving than in the foods on Levels 1 or 2.

Fats, Oils, and Sweets were put at the tip of the Pyramid because it's appropriately the smallest section. You'll notice there is no serving recommendation, only the admonition to eat and use these items "sparingly." The shape of the Pyramid also makes sense if you try to imagine it turned upside down; that is, attempting to make fats, oils, and sweets the "foundation." What would happen? It would teeter back and forth for a while, and then fall over, just as someone who ate that way eventually would.

So, let's start climbing the Food Guide Pyramid, beginning at its real base.

Level 1: Bread, Cereal, Rice, and Pasta Group

The title of this group is fairly descriptive. It includes such starchy foods as bread, rice, pasta, dry cereal, cooked cereal, crackers, rolls, bulgur wheat, tortillas, popcorn, pretzels, and rice cakes. Cake, cookies, and doughnuts, which are made with flour and, therefore, contain the same nutrients, are legitimately part of this group, but are actually more like "sweets," which are in the tip of the Pyramid. Most of the other items in this group are much better sources of nutrition and do not burden us with the extra fat and sugar contained in baked goods.

Foods in the Bread, Cereal, Rice, and Pasta Group provide a variety of nutrients, but contain very little protein, calcium, vitamin A, vitamin C, or folic acid. We have to get these nutrients from other parts of the Pyramid. This group's major nutrition contributions are:

- Carbohydrates, a major source of energy for all body functions
- B vitamins, to help us metabolize our food properly
- Fiber, for digestion and decreased risk of many serious diseases

Since this is the largest portion of the Pyramid, your child should get six to eleven servings from this level. This may sound like a lot, but serving sizes aren't as big as you might think, and they vary by age. See the chart on page 105 for suggested serving sizes for each of the food groups for children of different ages.

When it comes to serving size, we're not talking about the amount you actually serve, but specific, nutrition-related amounts of the various types of food in a group. For example, for a four-year-old, serving sizes include:

- one slice of bread—if you make a sandwich with two slices, that's two servings
- a half cup of dry cereal—maybe your child eats closer to a cup of cereal
- a third of a cup of cooked noodles or rice—measure it out and see how small it is

For optimal nutrition from this group, try to pick whole grains for the extra mineral and higher fiber content they provide, compared to items made from white flour. But if your child doesn't like whole wheat bread, don't panic or force it. White bread has the same amount of carbohydrate and is enriched with many of the same vitamins and minerals as whole wheat bread. When possible, try to find whole grains your family likes. Corn tortillas, whole wheat crackers, and rye bread are whole grains they might enjoy.

One of the extra benefits about this food group is that most of the items listed here do not have much fat. But beware. While it's true that most starches aren't high in fat, they can be fattening if you eat too much of them. And they become even more fattening if you put toppings like butter, margarine, or cream cheese on them. Also, watch out for items in this group such as muffins and some crackers, which may contain more fat than you think. Look for low-fat and fat-free crackers instead of high-fat ones, and make your own low-fat muffins. And as we said, some sweets are "officially" in this food group. However, a cookie might have some of the same vitamins as a piece of bread, but it comes along with a lot of unwanted fat and/or sugar.

Level 2: Vegetable Group

Although it's on the same level as the Fruit Group, the Vegetable Group is larger and was placed first on the row to indicate the greater nutritional contributions of vegetables. The group includes all vegetables, including starchy ones like potatoes and corn.

Vegetables contain very little protein and are not good sources of B vitamins. However, some of the dark green vegetables, such as broccoli and spinach, do have significant amounts of calcium, though not as much as items in the Milk, Yogurt, and Cheese Group. The main contributions from the Vegetable Group include:

- Vitamin A, for good eyesight, to keep skin healthy, and promote growth and wound healing
- Vitamin C, essential for tissue building and wound healing
- Folic Acid, for healthy red blood cells

Vegetables also can contribute fiber and some minerals, such as iron.

While it is relatively easy to ensure that children eat the six to eleven servings from the Bread, Cereal, Rice, and Pasta Group, it may be more challenging to get your child to eat three to five servings of vegetables a day. It helps that serving sizes are smaller for younger children and become larger only with age. For example, for four- to six-year-olds, a third of a cup of vegetables counts for a serving; while for seven- to ten-year-olds, it's a half cup.

The good news is that the Vegetable Group is a great place to give children second helpings if they're still hungry. This only works when you serve vegetables they like. Vegetables are good filler foods, providing lots of nutrients and bulk for relatively few calories. So for most vegetables, don't be concerned about serving size. The only exceptions are the starchy vegetables, such as potatoes and corn. Although they are classified as vegetables, they possess the same amount of carbohydrates and calories as foods in the Bread, Cereal,

Rice, and Pasta Group. So if you're serving a starchy vegetable at a meal, it's a good idea to balance it with a nonstarchy one, for example, potatoes and green beans, or corn-on-the-cob and broccoli.

The most important objective in choosing from the Vegetable Group is to find a variety of vegetables your child will eat. But for greatest nutritional impact try to pick ones that are high in vitamin A (beta-carotene) or vitamin C. Here are some good sources of these important nutrients:

- Vitamin C: broccoli, Brussels sprouts, cauliflower, kale, tomatoes, spinach, sweet red pepper
- Vitamin A: broccoli, carrots, collard greens, kale, spinach, sweet potatoes, winter squash
- Folic Acid: asparagus, black-eyed peas, broccoli, peas, romaine lettuce, spinach, sweet potatoes

Vegetables are good either raw or cooked. So if your child doesn't like cooked vegetables, give him raw veggies with a low-fat dip or slice them up in salads. If he doesn't care for raw vegetables, try cooking them. Fresh or frozen vegetables can be steamed until they're just tender-crisp or cooked in a small amount of water to retain as many vitamins as possible. Many frozen vegetables can be cooked in the microwave with no added water. Another great vegetable option is vegetables in soup.

One last point about vegetable nutrition: Fresh is generally better than frozen; and frozen is better than canned, especially if the canned vegetables contain added salt.

Level 2: Fruit Group

As its name indicates, the Fruit Group includes fruit—all fruit, from avocados to watermelons. Yes, avocados are fruits. But they're the black sheep of the fruit family because they are the only high-fat fruit in the basket. So if we had our way, we would put avocados in the tip of the Pyramid to indicate that they should be eaten sparingly, like other fats.

Fruits contain no protein or calcium and negligible amounts of the B vitamins. What they do offer are the same nutrients as many vegetables: vitamin A, vitamin C, and folic acid, along with fiber.

The recommended amount of fruit is two to four servings a day. For optimal nutrition, have a variety of fruits available to your child. The following are the best sources for vitamins A and C and folic acid:

- Vitamin A: apricots, cantaloupe, mango, papaya
- Vitamin C: cantaloupe, cranberry juice, grapefruit, honeydew melon, kiwi fruit, mango, oranges, orange juice, papaya, and strawberries
- Folic Acid: cantaloupe, oranges, orange juice, pineapple juice, plaintain

As with vegetables, fresh fruit is better than canned. But if your child will eat only canned or you can't get good fresh fruit during some months of the year, buy fruit canned in its own juice. And if it is only available in syrup, choose light syrup instead of heavy syrup. After all, canned peaches for dessert are lower in fat and calories and higher in nutrition than a cupcake.

Level 3: Milk, Yogurt, and Cheese Group

The food in this group includes every kind of milk (fat-free, low-fat, whole, even chocolate), all kinds of cheese, and every kind of yogurt (fat-free, low-fat, plain, flavored, and frozen). It also includes cream and ice cream.

These dairy products contain negligible amounts of vitamin C and fiber. However, most are excellent sources of the nutrients responsible for building and maintaining strong bones and teeth and creating new tissue. These include calcium, protein, and vitamins A and D (because milk products are fortified with these vitamins). It's important to note that the protein provided by the foods in this group is as good quality as the protein found in meat, poultry, and fish.

The recommendation for children is three servings from the Milk, Yogurt, and Cheese Group. The goal here is to provide the greatest amount of calcium for the least amount of fat. And, although the foods in this group seem quite similar, they vary widely in terms of calories, fat, and calcium per serving.

For example, whole milk, 2 percent, 1 percent, and fat-free milk all have the same amount of calcium, but the whole milk has double the calories and twenty times more fat than fat-free milk.

Serving sizes in this group are also a bit tricky. For example, for a seven- to ten-year-old, one cup (eight ounces) of fat-free milk is a serving, as is one and a half ounces of American cheese, because they both contribute about the same amount of protein and calcium. The glass of milk seems much larger, but it actually has about half of the calories and 65 percent less fat than the cheese.

And when you see the serving size for cheese, don't consider the same amount of cottage cheese as equal in nutrition. It would take one and a half cups (12 ounces) of cottage cheese to equal the calcium of one and a half ounces of regular cheese. However, cottage cheese does have the advantage of being lower in fat and higher in protein.

In addition to calcium, the other nutritional consideration in this group is fat. But in the case of fat, you want less of it rather than more. When it comes to milk or yogurt, try to use reduced-fat or fat-free varieties. Most cheeses are high in fat, but there are a wide variety of reduced-fat cheeses that your children will probably like. Fat-free cheese is another option, but not if they won't eat it.

Ice cream is one of the highest-fat and least nutritious items in this group. Not only is it lower in protein than most of the other dairy products, but one would need to eat one and a half cups (nearly a whole pint) of ice cream to equal the calcium in a cup of 2% milk. One and a half cups of ice cream can have between 450 and 900 calories, compared to 125 calories for one cup of 2% milk; and ice cream derives 50 to 70 percent of those calories from fat, while the milk gets just 36 percent from fat.

Level 3: Meat, Poultry, Fish, Dry Beans, Eggs, and Nuts Group

This group includes meat, such as lamb, beef, and pork; poultry, such as chicken and turkey; eggs; all kinds of fish and shellfish; dry beans, including soybean products like tofu; legumes, such as lentils; and all varieties of nuts.

What do the foods in this diverse group have in common? They are the richest sources of protein, iron, selenium, and zinc in the diet. Although these foods contain negligible vitamin A and vitamin C, and just a few B vitamins, they provide protein for growth, effective wound healing, and healthy blood. In addition, they contain significant amounts of niacin, which also supports these vital functions of the body.

Given the importance of the nutrients provided by the foods in this group, you may think that two to three servings a day isn't enough. Since just 15 percent of a child's calorie intake needs to come from protein, the servings and serving sizes are more than adequate.

In this group, the serving sizes are more uniform than in the Milk, Yogurt, and Cheese Group. An ounce of beef, chicken, and fish and one egg all provide approximately the same amount of protein and iron. However, the fat content varies significantly among them. Check back to The Big Picture of Fat on page 89 to see how much they vary. Beans and legumes have the least amount of fat, but you have to eat more of them to get equal amounts of protein. Nuts are the highest fat items in this group, so high that they shouldn't be used routinely as sources of protein, but rather as treats. The exception to the rule is peanut butter, because it's such a favorite for children. On days when your child has a peanut butter and jelly sandwich, you can balance it with a variety of lower-fat foods.

Because the nutrient content is so consistent throughout this group, for optimal nutrition try to choose those items lower in fat. We'll help you identify them in the next chapter.

Level 4: Fats, Oils, and Sweets

Displaying sweets and fats at the pinnacle of the Pyramid doesn't mean they are the best. Rather, because the top of a pyramid is the smallest part, it conveys that sweets and fats should contribute the smallest percentage of one's food intake. This is the place reserved for foods with nothing to offer except fat or sugar. Notable in this category are oil, butter, mayonnaise, margarine, cream cheese, bacon, olives, whipping cream, candy, and soda.

All but the last two items we mentioned in this category are roughly equal in fat: they derive all, or almost all, of their calories from fat. Candy can contain just sugar and no fat (hard candies, licorice, or jelly beans) or it can be high in both sugar and fat (chocolate and other creamy candies).

The key to foods in this category is to offer them infrequently and in moderation. This is the category that most "treats" come from, which is okay as long as the treats are not everyday occurrences or served in excessive amounts.

Beverages

Remember, we said that water is one of the most important nutrients for health. In fact, children should drink about six to eight glasses of fluids a day. Milk, juices, soup, and other liquids can be counted as part of the daily requirement.

Most parents know to limit the amount of soda pop children drink on a daily basis, but may give carte blanche to fruit juice because it seems healthier. However, even though fruit juice is listed in the Fruit Group, there's a big difference between juice and the fruit it's squeezed from. The truth is, nutritionally, most fruit juice is just like soda without the bubbles.

When it comes to nutrients, not all juices are created equal. Only a few are good sources of vitamin C, such as orange, grapefruit, cranberry, tomato, and those "fortified" with vitamin C. However, apple and grape, two of the most popular juices for children, contain only a trace of this essential vitamin.

As for fiber, no juice stacks up to its "real fruit" counterpart. For example, apples have three times the fiber of apple juice, and an orange has eight times the fiber of its juice.

So what is your child getting in a glass or box of apple juice? No nutrients, no fiber—just sugar. Furthermore, many children drink more than one cup of juice a day. In fact, frequent trips to the refrigerator can easily add up to 500 empty calories, the equivalent of nearly four cans of soda per day.

Juice is also a fraud when it purports to be as healthy a thirst quencher as milk, because juice has none of milk's vital nutrients, such as calcium, protein, and vitamins A and D. So if children are allowed to substitute juice for milk, they're missing out on a lot of good nutrition—unless you're buying calcium-fortified juice.

What can you do if your child is a soda or juice fanatic? In either case, encourage her to drink reduced-fat milk with meals and snacks and water in between when she's thirsty.

For the times when only soda will do, it's better for your child to have a diet soda than to ingest all of the sugar and calories in a regular soda. And while parents may be concerned about the aspartame sweetener in diet soda, the FDA has concluded that aspartame is safe for the general public, including children. However, you should be alert to the caffeine in many sodas, and choose those that are caffeine-free.

Serving Sizes for Different-Age Children

Age	2–3 Years	4–6 Years	7 and Up
Breads/Grains (6–11 servings)			
Bread	¹/₂ slice	1 slice	1 slice
Cooked cereal	¹/₄–¹/₃ cup	¹/₃–¹/₂cup	¹/₂ cup
Dry cereal	¹/₂ ounce	¹/₂–³/₄ ounce	1 ounce
Pasta/rice	¹/₄–¹/₃ cup	¹/₃–¹/₂ cup	¹/₂ cup
Vegetables (3–5 servings)			
Cooked/raw	2–3 TBS	¹/₃ cup	¹/₂ cup
Salad greens	¹/₄ cup	¹/₂ cup	1 cup
Fruits (2–4 servings)			
Canned/cut up	2–3 TBS	¹/₃ cup	¹/₂ cup
Fresh fruit	¹/₄–¹/₂ small piece	¹/₂–1 small piece	1 piece
Juice	¹/₄–¹/₃ cup	¹/₂ cup	³/₄ cup
Dried	not recommended due to choking risk	3 TBS	¹/₄ cup
Milk products (2–3 servings)			
Milk	1 cup	1 cup	1 cup
Cheese	1 ounce	1¹/₂ ounces	1¹/₂–2 ounces
Yogurt	1 cup	1 cup	1 cup
Fish, Poultry, Meat, Beans, Nuts, and Eggs (2–3 servings)			
Fish, poultry, meat (cooked)	¹/₂–1 ounce	1¹/₂ ounces	2¹/₂–3 ounces
Dry beans (cooked)	¹/₃ cup	¹/₂ cup	1–1¹/₂ cups
Peanut butter	1 TBS	1–2 TBS	2–3 TBS
Eggs	1	1	2

For the juice fan, make a special place for fruit juice at breakfast or lunch, and choose one that's high in vitamin C. For snacks, offer fresh fruit instead of juice. If it's hard cutting back, try watering down her favorite flavors—that way she'll only be getting half the sugar. Or pour milk for the first glass and juice for the second.

Does this sound like a lot of food for your child? It really isn't, considering the fact that it's for the whole day and should be spread out over three meals and two to three snacks. Also, keep in mind that while the younger children in each age category should eat at least the minimum number of servings indicated, older children probably will be closer to the top of the range. In the next chapter, we'll give you some sample menus to show you how it can work.

13

Healthy Choices
on Each Level

ARE YOU READY TO CLIMB the Food Guide Pyramid again? In the last chapter we examined the nutrients available on each level, but this time we're going to go up the Pyramid with a special focus on fat and calories. The object is to show you how to keep the nutrients essential for your child's health and growth, while losing some of the unnecessary fat and sugar that may be contributing to her being overweight.

As you read this chapter, you may want to refer back to the Food Records you filled out in chapter 4. By the end of this chapter, you'll be able to figure out how many servings from each food group your child ate on the days you recorded, as well as which items were high in fat and sugar.

But first, let's look at scenarios of three children's eating habits. These scenarios are one-day snapshots that represent each child's customary pattern of eating.

Teresa's Trouble Spots

Teresa is a fourteen-year-old who is responsible for her own breakfast and lunch. Her parents give her money for lunch, and she has a weekend job, so she can buy pretty much whatever she feels like eating. On this Thursday morning, there's food at home for her to make breakfast, but since she's running late, she picks up apple juice, a doughnut, and a bag of chips at the corner market near her school. She eats the doughnut and drinks the juice on her way to homeroom.

In between two of her morning classes, she munches on the bag of chips. Her lunch from the cafeteria line consists of a hamburger, fries, and a large Coke. When she gets home from school, she scoops up a bowl of ice cream to tide her over until dinnertime. At dinner, her mom has fixed meatloaf, potatoes au gratin, spinach, and bread, but Teresa skips the spinach. Later, while she's studying, she munches on a chocolate candy bar.

How do you think Teresa's day stacks up on the Pyramid? See page 109.

Evaluation: Teresa's food intake was high in fat and sugar and low in nutrition. Of particular concern is the virtual lack of dairy products. And although it might look as though she got four of the minimum five vegetables and fruits, they aren't particularly good choices—her potatoes all have more fat than nutrition and the apple juice is mostly sugar. It was difficult for Teresa to even get enough servings from the Grain Group.

Good Intentions Miss the Mark

Eleven-year-old Mark's parents are knowledgeable about good nutrition for their son and have tried to teach him some of the principles. However, they have always ignored the fat and sugar that comes along with the nutrients. On this Friday morning, Mark has breakfast at home: sugar-coated flakes with a banana and whole milk, and a glass of orange juice. Since he didn't bring a mid-morning snack to school, he's starving by lunch and buys two hot dogs, a carton of 2% milk, and an apple. At home after school, he finds a package of chocolate cupcakes and a glass of whole milk. Then, for dinner, he eats salad with ranch dressing, a pork chop, some buttered mixed vegetables, two pieces of corn bread with more butter, and three cookies. While watching a movie with his family, he shares in the buttered microwave popcorn, along with an orange soda. See Mark's chart on page 110.

Teresa's Day

Food Group	Recommended Servings	Teresa's Servings	Foods	Comments
Oils, Sweets	Sparingly	2	Coke Candy bar	Both high in sugar and empty calories, candy bar high in fat
Dairy	2–3	1	Ice cream	Technically in the dairy group, ice cream is lower in calcium and protein than other choices and higher in fat and sugar
Meats	2–3	2	Hamburger Meatloaf	Higher fat, 2 red meats in one day
Vegetables	3–5	3	Potato chips French fries Potatoes au gratin	All high fat, no vitamin A or folic acid sources
Fruits	2–4	1	Apple juice	Low nutrition, high in sugar
Grains	6–11	4	Doughnut Hamburger bun Bread	Doughnut is high fat/high sugar, no whole grains

Mark's Day

Food Group	Recommended Servings	Mark's Servings	Foods	Comments
Oils, Sweets	Sparingly	4	Soda Butter on mixed vegetables, cornbread, and popcorn	Soda high in sugar. Lots of added fat
Dairy	2–3	3	Whole milk (2) 2% milk	Both are equally good sources of calcium, but whole milk is higher in fat
Meats	2–3	2	Hot dogs (2) Pork chop	Both high-fat meats
Vegetables	3–5	2	Salad with ranch dressing Mixed vegetables	Ranch dressing is high in fat, butter added extra fat to vegetables
Fruits	2–4	3	Apple juice Orange juice Apple	Good choices
Grains	6–11	11	Sugar-coated flakes Hot dog buns (2) Cookies (3) Cupcakes (2) Corn bread (2) Microwave popcorn	Cereal high in sugar; cookies, cupcakes high in fat and sugar; corn bread high in fat; popcorn medium fat

Evaluation: Mark's daily diet covers all the nutritional bases quite well, but too many of the choices are high in fat and/or sugar.

Debbie's Dilemma

Debbie is a five-year-old whose parents are overly concerned about fat. Her mother is always on a diet to keep her weight under control, and her father has a high cholesterol level, so he's focused on keeping his fat intake down, too. For breakfast, her mom gives Debbie a piece of toast with jelly and a glass of grape juice. Debbie doesn't like milk, and her mother says that juice is okay as a substitute because she thinks it's as healthy as fruit. While they're out doing errands in the car this Saturday morning, Debbie munches on a bagel. For lunch, they stop for a turkey sandwich and apple juice. In the afternoon, Debbie gets to have some frozen yogurt as a snack. For dinner, it's pasta with marinara sauce, salad with fat-free dressing, French bread, and a popsicle for dessert.

Debbie's diet is certainly low in fat, but what else is it low in? See page 112.

Evaluation: By focusing too much on keeping Debbie's diet low in fat, her parents are not providing adequate nutrition for her growth. Particularly distressing is the virtual lack of dairy products and the skimpy servings from the Meat, Vegetable, and Fruit Groups.

If these Food Records of Teresa, Mark, and Debbie represented just one day in an otherwise healthy food week, there would be no cause for concern. However, if these days are typical of the entire week, there's a lot of room for improvement. If your child's Four-Day Food Records resemble any of these scenarios, our suggestions will help you find ways to increase the nutrition and/or lower the fat and sugar.

Each of the next sections details one of the food groups in the Pyramid and provides examples of low-, medium- and high-fat food choices in the group. We suggest that you think of these categories not in terms of how many grams of fat the food items have, or the percentage of calories from fat, but rather in a more functional way.

- *Low-fat* items are the ones your child can have *every day*. These should form the major component of his or her daily or weekly food intake. The exceptions are low-fat foods that are very high in sugar. These should be eaten in moderation because of their high calorie content.

Debbie's Day

Food Group	Recommended Servings	Debbie's Servings	Foods	Comments
Oils, Sweets	Sparingly	1	Popsicle	Empty calories
Dairy	2–3	1	Frozen yogurt	Technically a choice from the dairy group, but it's low in calcium and high in sugar
Meats	2–3	1	Turkey	Good low-fat meat, but short of the recommended 2 servings
Vegetables	3–5	1	Salad	Not enough vegetables
Fruits	2–4	2	Grape juice Apple juice	Low-nutrition fruit choices—mostly sugar
Grains	6–11	7	Toast Bagel (counts as 2 servings) Bread for sandwich Pasta Bread	Lots of grains, with no added fat

- *Medium-fat* items are ones that are best used in *moderation*. Depending upon your child's food preferences, it will be okay to include some foods in this category each day in order to provide good nutrition and variety.
- *High-fat* items should be targeted for use *only occasionally*, not just because they are high in fat, but because they often are high in sugar and low in nutrition as well.

Each food group has different nutrition, calorie, and fat challenges, so we'll address them separately.

Bread, Cereal, Rice, and Pasta Group

The good news is that there are lots of low-fat choices in the Bread, Cereal, Rice, and Pasta Group. The bad news is that they can easily be transformed into high-fat items. Take bread, for example. A slice of whole wheat toast has about 75 calories and negligible fat. But if you add just one teaspoon of butter or margarine to that same slice of toast, you've turned it into a high-fat food with 120 calories, 38 percent from fat. The same is true for rice, a good low-fat food that can become a high-fat item when it's made into fried rice.

And be aware that a number of dry cereals are high in sugar. Compare the labels of the cereals your child likes and choose those with the fewest grams of sugar per serving. Every 5 grams is equivalent to a teaspoon of sugar.

Try to encourage your child to eat a couple of servings of whole-grain items from this group, to get the fiber and added minerals that whole grains provide. Choices include whole-grain breads, crackers, or pasta, as well as brown rice and many breakfast cereals.

You'll notice that cookies and other sweets are listed in this group. And even though there are a lot of low-fat sweets on the store shelves, most are laden with sugar. This means that they can still be quite high in calories and are best eaten in smaller quantities. Nonetheless, they are better choices than cookies high in both sugar and fat. And when eaten in moderation, these low-fat sweets provide reasonable treats for children.

Vegetable Group

Vegetables are naturally low in fat and high in fiber, so it's hard to go wrong in this group. Since variety is the key, try to help your child find as many different vegetables as possible that he likes. In addition to the old standards—iceberg lettuce and mixed vegetables—offer him some dark-green vegetables, such as spinach, romaine lettuce, and broccoli; deep-yellow vegetables, such as carrots and sweet potatoes; and legumes, such as kidney beans and garbanzo beans.

Starchy vegetables, such as corn, peas, lima beans, and potatoes, are good choices, too. But remember, although they contain no fat, their calorie and starch content is similar to foods in the Bread Group.

Bread, Cereal, Rice, and Pasta Group

Low-Fat	Medium-Fat	High-Fat
• most bread and rolls • English muffins • bagels • hamburger and hot dog buns • pita bread • plain tortillas	• most breadsticks	• biscuits • bread stuffing • corn bread • fried tortilla or taco shells
• low-sugar dry cereal • high-sugar dry cereal* • cooked cereal • low-fat or fat-free granola cereal*	• most waffles, pancakes, and French toast • items made with biscuit mix	• regular granola cereal* • doughnuts* • scones* • muffins*
• rice—white or brown • pasta noodles • couscous • grits • polenta • Kashi	• some packaged rice and noodle mixes	• fried rice • some packaged rice and noodle mixes • chow mein noodles
• low-fat or fat-free crackers • pretzels • air-popped popcorn • rice cakes • some "light" microwave popcorn • fat-free caramel corn*	• some "light" microwave popcorn	• traditional snack crackers • cheese crackers, puffs, and curls • corn chips • corn nuts • tortilla chips • nacho chips • regular popcorn • regular caramel corn*
• graham crackers* • animal crackers* • ginger snaps* • fig newtons and other newtons* • low-fat or fat-free cookies and cakes* • low-fat or fat-free granola bars* • plain angel food cake*	• some cookies*	• many cookies* • brownies* • cake* • cupcakes* • pastry* • pie crust • regular granola bars*

*Usually contain a lot of sugar and are likely to be high in calories.

In order to work toward the minimum three servings a day from the Vegetable Group, get creative: Include raw vegetables as snacks, and try serving cooked vegetable salads (such as three-bean salad) or putting vegetables in soups and stews.

Since vegetables contain no fat and so few calories in their natural state, the only way they become high-fat or even medium-fat foods is when we add toppings or cook them in butter or rich sauces. See below for examples.

Vegetable Group

Low-Fat	Medium-Fat	High-Fat
All vegetables—when nothing is added to them other than seasonings; fat-free mayonnaise, margarine, or sour cream; or plain fat-free or low-fat yogurt	Vegetables with low-fat toppings, such as reduced-fat salad dressings, low-fat sour cream, reduced-fat mayonnaise, light margarine	Vegetables with high-fat toppings, such as regular salad dressing, oil, mayonnaise, butter, margarine, cheese sauce, or cream sauce
Vegetable juices		Cole slaw Potato salad Fried vegetables, such as French fries and onion rings
Sources of vitamin A, vitamin C, and/or Folic Acid		
asparagus black-eyed peas broccoli Brussels sprouts carrots cauliflower collard greens kale peas romaine lettuce spinach sweet potatoes sweet red pepper tomatoes winter squash		

Fruit Group

Just like vegetables, fruits are naturally low in fat and calories. The only exceptions are avocados, coconut, and olives, which should be eaten sparingly. Otherwise, your child can enjoy all kinds of fruits.

The only concern in the Fruit Group is that the two to four servings a day do not rely too heavily on fruit juice or dried fruit. As we've said, most fruit juice is no better than soda because of its sugar content. The issue with dried fruits is that, without the water that exists in fresh fruit, they contain more sugar per ounce and, therefore, are higher in calories. An ounce of dried apricots has about 70 calories, whereas an ounce of fresh apricots contains just 15.

Fruit Group

Low-Fat	Medium-Fat	High-Fat
All fruits except the three in the high-fat column		Avocado Olives Coconut
Dried fruit* Fruit juices		Fruit pies and cobblers* Fruit topped with whipped cream
Sources of vitamin A, vitamin C, and/or Folic Acid		
apricots cantaloupe cranberry juice grapefruit honeydew melon kiwi fruit mango oranges orange juice papaya pineapple juice plantain strawberries		

*Usually contain a lot of sugar and are likely to be high in calories.

Milk, Yogurt, and Cheese Group

In the Milk, Yogurt, and Cheese Group there are many choices at every fat level. The key is to find lower-fat dairy products that your child enjoys. If you try to change from a high-fat item, such as whole milk, to a lower-fat choice, such as 2% or 1% milk, you'll be more successful if you do it gradually. We'll help you with these kinds of issues in chapter 15, where we focus on fat-lowering strategies.

Milk, Yogurt, and Cheese Group

Low-Fat	Medium-Fat	High-Fat
• fat-free milk • fat-free evaporated milk • 1% milk • fat-free chocolate milk* • fat-free buttermilk • fat-free cream substitutes	• 2% milk • evaporated low-fat milk • low-fat chocolate milk* • low-fat buttermilk	• whole milk • evaporated whole milk • buttermilk cultured from whole milk • half-and-half • whipping cream • cream substitutes
• fat-free yogurt • low-fat yogurt		• whole-milk yogurt
• fat-free and low-fat cottage cheese • fat-free cheeses • fat-free cream cheese	• part-skim mozzarella cheese • part-skim ricotta cheese • string cheese • many "reduced-fat" cheeses	• most cheses including Brie, Edam, feta, cream cheese, whole-milk mozzarella, Parmesan, Swiss, cheddar, American, Monterey Jack
• fat-free sour cream	• reduced-fat or "light" sour cream	• sour cream
• fat-free frozen yogurt* • fat-free ice cream* • some low-fat frozen yogurts* • some light ice creams* • fat-free puddings and pudding made with fat-free milk* • pudding pops*	• some frozen yogurts* • some "light" ice creams* • puddings made with low-fat milk*	• ice cream* • whole-milk puddings*

*Usually contain a lot of sugar and are likely to be high in calories.

Also, it's important to realize that some low-fat dairy products are high in sugar, particularly frozen yogurt and light ice creams. This makes them higher in calories than some of the other choices in the low-fat column.

What if your child is allergic to milk? If lactose is a problem, you can try lactose-reduced, low-fat milk products. There are also brands of low-fat soy milk. But you need to buy one with added calcium in order to provide a good substitute for milk.

Meat, Poultry, Fish, Dry Beans, Eggs, and Nuts Group

Most Americans, children included, eat more from this food group than they need for good nutrition. Although we may eat from this group just two times a day, our portion sizes tend to be larger than the recommended serving size of two to three ounces.

Although there are a number of good low-fat choices in this group, it's weighted more heavily toward medium- and high-fat protein sources. One strategy for minimizing the fat is to cook and serve smaller

Meat, Poultry, Fish, Dry Beans, Eggs, and Nuts Group

Low-Fat	Medium-Fat	High-Fat
• cooked dried beans, peas, and lentils • lentil or bean soup	• tofu	• nuts • peanut and other nut butters
• egg whites		• whole eggs
• shellfish • most other fish • water-pack tuna	• some fish (salmon, tuna in oil)	• breaded, fried fish, including fish sticks
• white-meat chicken and turkey (skinless)	• dark-meat chicken and turkey (skinless)	• chicken and turkey with skin • fried chicken
• top round steak (London broil) • eye of the round roast • liver	• leanest ground beef • veal • some pork (center loin) • tripe	• most beef • most lamb • most pork • spare ribs • chitterlings
• low-fat lunchmeat • low-fat hot dogs	• extra-lean ham	• cold cuts (bologna, salami, ham) • hot dogs • bacon • sausage

amounts of meat, fish, and poultry. A three-ounce serving of meat is about the size of a deck of cards or a medium chicken-breast half.

Also, it's good to aim for no more than three to four servings of red meat a week—that naturally helps keep the fat down. And choosing nonmeat protein sources from the low-fat column a couple of times a week will help, too.

Fats, Oils, and Sweets

This is the "use sparingly" group. The easiest way to cut down in this group is to avoid adding fat to foods without thinking—maybe they don't need it. For example, you may be in the habit of putting a pat of butter on the green beans, but they may taste just as good with some fresh herbs.

Fats, Oils, and Sweets Group

Low-Fat	Medium-Fat	High-Fat
• *fat-free* dressings, mayonnaise, margarine, sour creams, etc.	• *reduced-fat* salad dressings and mayonnaise • Diet or light margarine	• all *regular* fats including all oil mayonnaise, margarine, butter • regular salad dressings • bacon
• sugar-type candy: jelly beans, gum drops, gummy bears, Lifesavers* • marshmallows* • licorice*	• some chocolate-covered mint patties* • Tootsie Rolls, Tootsie Roll Pops* • chewy honey candy*	• chocolate candy* • candy with nuts*
• jellies and jams* • pancake syrup* • chocolate syrup*		• chocolate fudge sauces*
• fruit gelatin* • juice bars* • Popsicles*		
• diet soda • soda water, mineral water, seltzer • soda* • fruit punch* • Kool-Aid* • sports drinks*		• milkshakes* • commercial fruit smoothies*

*Usually contain a lot of sugar and are likely to be high in calories.

Also, if you try to help your child eat fewer items from this group, you may want to introduce the concept of prioritizing fats and sweets. This means making a conscious choice of which high-fat, high-sugar foods he can't do without, instead of eating them simply out of habit or because they're available.

And don't overlook soda, juice drinks, fruit punch, and other high-sugar drinks, which can quickly add empty calories. For example, one 12-ounce can of soda has 150 calories, equal to 7½ teaspoons of sugar—with zero nutritional value. And even worse, most children who drink soda drink much more than one can per day. If your child is hooked on soda, try cutting down and/or substituting soda water mixed with fruit juice or diet soda in moderation.

Another strategy is to replace higher-fat items with lower-fat ones. Fortunately, there are dozens of lower-fat spreads, dressings, and condiments. We'll show you how to spot the really low-fat ones when we take a tour of the supermarket.

Low-Fat Cooking Tips

The way you prepare and cook foods will do one of three things to their fat content.

1. Increase the fat by adding oil, butter, margarine, cream, etc., to low-fat foods.
2. Reduce the fat by using cooking techniques that remove extra fat.
3. Keep the fat low by using low-fat or fat-free preparation and cooking methods.

For obvious reasons we're going to focus on the last two approaches.

Trimming the Fat

- Broiling or grilling meats lets some of the fat drip away while they cook. Be sure to coat the pan or grill with vegetable oil spray to keep the meat from sticking.
- Roasting meats and poultry on a rack in a broiler pan also allows some of the fat to cook out. For easy cleanup, line the broiler pan with aluminum foil.
- Braising or stewing foods slowly in a small amount of low-fat liquid works well when slow cooking is required. And if you

prepare the dish ahead of time, you can refrigerate it overnight to allow the fat from the meat to congeal on the top. Then just skim off and discard the hardened fat before reheating. This defatting technique also works for soups and stocks.

- If you can't prepare stews or soups in advance, reduce the fat by skimming off as much of it as possible and adding several ice cubes to the warm liquid. The fat will cling to the ice, which can be quickly removed and discarded.
- Brown ground meat in a nonstick skillet. After cooking, spoon the cooked meat into a colander to drain excess fat. If you want to get rid of even more fat, rinse the ground meat with hot water and pat it dry with paper towels after draining. If meat and other ingredients are to be added back to the skillet, wipe drippings from pan with a paper towel.
- Trim all visible fat from meat and remove the skin and visible fat from poultry before cooking.

Keeping Foods Low in Fat

- Poaching in broth, or some other nonfat liquid, is a great way to cook chicken or fish while keeping them moist and juicy.
- Steaming is a nonfat way to cook vegetables while retaining their vitamins and minerals. It's also good for fish.
- Baking is another fat-free cooking technique that's good for meat, poultry, and fish.
- Stir-frying or sautéing in a nonstick skillet or wok sprayed with vegetable spray is good for cooking meat or vegetables quickly.
- Foods that are cooked in a microwave oven generally require little or no added fat. Most suitable for microwaving are those foods with a high moisture content, such as vegetables, fruits, fish, and sauces.
- Coat baking dishes, pans, and casseroles with vegetable cooking spray instead of butter, oil, or shortening. You can flour a sprayed baking pan just as you would if it were "greased" the high-fat way.
- Marinate lean meats, fish, and poultry in fat-free or low-fat marinades to enhance flavors. Reduce or omit oil from marinade recipes by substituting water, broth, or wine (the alcohol cooks away). Other low-fat ingredients for marinades include citrus juices and flavored vinegars.

Substituting for Maximum Flavor and Minimum Fat

Another way to trim the fat in cooking is to substitute items that are lower in fat than some of the ingredients called for in your favorite recipes. These substitutions won't work for all recipes. You will have to experiment to make sure that you aren't losing flavor or texture while you cut out some of the fat. In general, the *lower*-fat substitutions are less conspicuous than fat-free options, so you may want to try them first. And if the recipe just doesn't work with a low-fat alternative, try using a smaller amount of the high-fat ingredient.

If the recipe calls for a high-fat ingredient	Try a lower fat substitute	If it works, use a nonfat substitute
butter or margarine	reduced-fat margarine	fat-free spreads, vegetable oil spray, imitation butter sprinkles
oil for cooking and frying	reduced-fat margarine	broth, wine, juice, vegetable oil spray
cream cheese	light cream cheese	fat-free cream cheese product
sour cream	"light" sour cream	fat-free sour cream or fat-free or low-fat yogurt
2 eggs	1 whole egg plus 2 egg whites	4 egg whites or equivalent egg substitute
mayonnaise	reduced-calorie mayonnaise	fat-free mayonnaise
salad dressing	reduced-calorie salad dressing	oil-free salad dressing
cream	milk	evaporated skimmed milk
chocolate, unsweetened	3 tablespoons unsweetened cocoa plus 1 tablespoon oil or margarine	

The Pyramid and Your Child

Now it's time to evaluate your child's Food Records from chapter 4. First, go through each day and tally the number of servings from each of the Food Groups. See the sample below for eight-year-old Michael. To help us tally, we've marked foods as *G* for the Grain Group; *V* for Vegetables; *F* for Fruits; *D* for dairy products; and *M* for the Meat Group. You will also want to make note of any vegetables or fruits that are good sources of vitamins A, C and/or folic acid (see pages 115–16).

	Time	Food and Beverages	Location	Comments
Breakfast	7:30 A.M.	*Chocolate puff cereal (G) With whole milk (D)*	*Kitchen*	*Helps himself*
Snacks	10 A.M.	*4 snack crackers (G) and 1 slice of American cheese (½ D) 1 glass apple juice (F)*	*Family room*	*Hungry*
Lunch	Noon	*Peanut butter (M) and jelly sandwich on white bread (2G) Handful of potato chips Glass of grape juice (F) 2 chocolate chip cookies (G)*	*Kitchen*	*He's in a peanut butter & jelly rut*
Snacks	3:00 P.M.	*2 cups of apple juice (2F)*	*At Soccer practice*	
	4:00 P.M.	*ice cream cone, one scoop (¼ D, ½ G)*	*In car*	*Stopped on way home from practice*
Dinner	6:30 P.M.	*½ bowl of spaghetti (G) with meat sauce (M) 1 piece of bread (G) with butter 1 glass of whole milk (D) 2 chocolate chip cookies (G)*	*Kitchen*	*Didn't want all of his spaghetti, but insisted on dessert*
Snacks	8:30 P.M.	*Bowl of microwave popcorn (shared bag with sister) (G) 1 cup grape juice (F)*	*Living room*	*Watching TV*

Next, circle the foods in these groups that are from any high-fat column in this chapter, as well as those added fats and sweets (even low-fat ones) that belong in the tip of the Pyramid.

Summary of Michael's Day

Grains:	9½ servings
Vegetables:	0 servings
Fruits:	5 servings
Dairy Products:	2¾ servings
Meats:	2 servings
CIRCLES:	11 high-fat foods

The numbers tell a lot of the story: Michael did fine with the Grains, Milk, and Meat Groups. Although he had five fruits, you'll notice that they were all fruit juices (high in sugar and calories), and none was a good source of vitamin C. Also, Michael didn't have any vegetables at all this day. The other area of concern is the eleven circles: some were high-fat nutritious choices, such as milk, peanut butter, cheese, and meat. But many were high-fat, high-calorie foods that added no nutrition, such as cookies, ice cream, and potato chips.

There's lots of room for improvement in Michael's eating pattern—both in terms of lowering fat and improving nutrition. See pages 125–26 for what Michael's Food Record might look like after gradual changes over time.

Before	Improved	Strategies
Chocolate puff cereal (G) with whole milk (D)	Half chocolate puff cereal/half toasted rice cereal (G) with low-fat milk (D)	Mixed a high-sugar cereal with a low-sugar cereal to cut sugar in half. Switched from whole milk to low-fat milk.
4 snack crackers (G) and 1 slice of American cheese (½ D) 1 glass apple juice (F)	4 reduced-fat snack crackers (G) and 1 string cheese (½ D) Handful baby carrots (V) Water	Found lower-fat crackers and lower-fat cheese he liked. A good place to work in a vegetable.
Peanut butter (M) and jelly sandwich on white bread (2G) Handful of potato chips Glass of grape juice (F) 2 chocolate chip cookies (G)	Peanut butter (M) and jelly sandwich on white bread (2G) Handful of pretzels (½ G) Grapes (F) 1 glass low-fat milk (D) 1 chocolate chip cookie (½ G)	PB&J is his favorite and it has lots of nutrition. Pretzels are as crunchy as chips, with less fat. Grapes have less sugar than grape juice. 1 chocolate chip cookie is still a treat.
2 cups of apple juice (2F) Ice cream cone, one scoop (¼ D, ½ G)	1 cup orange juice (F) 1 cup water Frozen yogurt cone, one scoop (½ D, ½ G)	Orange juice has vitamin C, but 2 glasses are not needed. Michael likes frozen yogurt just as much as ice cream and it has more calcium.

Before	Improved	Strategies
¹/₂ bowl of spaghetti (G) with meat sauce (M) 1 piece of bread (G) with (butter) 1 glass of (milk)(D) 2 (chocolate chip) (cookies)(G)	Green salad with reduced-calorie dressing (V) ¹/₂ bowl of spaghetti (G) with meat sauce (M) 1 piece of bread (G) with (reduced-fat) (margarine) 1 glass of low-fat milk (D) 1 (chocolate chip) (cookie)(¹/₂ G)	Salad counts as a vegetable, reduced-calorie dressing keeps the fat down.
Bowl of (microwave) (popcorn)(shared bag with sister) (G) 1 cup grape juice (F)	Bowl of low-fat microwave popcorn (shared bag with sister) (G) 1 cup grape juice (F)	Low-fat microwave popcorn saves a lot of fat. He can keep his grape juice as a treat.
Grains: 9¹/₂ Vegetables: 0 Fruits: 5* Dairy Products: 2³/₄ Meats: 2 CIRCLES: 11 *no vitamin A, C, or folic acid	Grains: 9 Vegetables: 2** Fruits: 3*** Dairy Products: 4 Meats: 2 CIRCLES: 4 (some of the circles are lower in fat than in "before") **one vitamin A ***one vitamin C	By making a number of small changes, we were able to greatly reduce the fat and improve Michael's nutrition.

Note that we didn't have to eliminate favorite foods or treats to provide Michael with lower-fat nutrition. In the next chapter, we'll help you develop strategies specific to your own child.

14

Be Supermarket Savvy

WITH THE EXCEPTION OF JACK SPRAT, just about everyone loves fat. We all love sugar, too. Fat and sugar provide a lot of the flavor and pleasing texture in many of the foods we eat. They also contribute the bulk of the calories.

Ounce for ounce, fat contains more than twice the calories of either protein or carbohydrate. A gram of fat contains 9 calories, while a gram of either protein or carbohydrate has just 4 calories. The goal of this chapter and chapter 15, "Calorie-Lowering Strategies Especially for Kids," is to help you find the extra fat and sugar that lurk in your child's diet and identify strategies for gradually reducing the amount, without sacrificing taste or texture. And since many children, like adults, don't eat the recommended number of servings from the Vegetable, Fruit, and Milk Groups, we'll also help you with ideas for increasing low-calorie selections from these groups.

Start With Your Child's Food Record

In the last chapter, we asked you to analyze your child's Food Records, looking not only for overall nutrition (the number of servings from each food group) but also for fat sources. We asked you to circle nutritious high-fat foods, as well as any food from the tip of the Pyramid—those fats and sweets that deliver mostly empty calories.

Let's take a closer look at those circles. They are good targets for your calorie-lowering efforts. Use the spaces below to record the items you circled. Write down each food item and indicate the number of times your child had it during the four days you kept the Food Records. You also can write in items that your child generally eats but just happened not to choose on those four days.

High-Fat or High-Sugar/Low Nutrition

Pure fat (butter, mayonnaise, sour cream, salad dressings, bacon):

_____

High-fat sauces:_____

Sautéed or fried foods:_____

High-fat crackers or chips: _____

Baked goods (cookies, cakes, brownies, doughnuts, pie):_____

_____

Ice cream: _____

Candy: _____

Soda and other high-sugar drinks: _____

Other: _____

High-Fat/Good Nutrition

Whole milk: _____

High-fat cheese: _____

Peanut butter: _____

Nuts: _____

Red meat: _____

Whole eggs: _____

Sausages/lunch meats: _____

Other: _____

Are you beginning to see some patterns in the high-calorie foods your child eats? Perhaps his high-fat choices are spread among the various categories, but more likely they are clustered in a few areas. Maybe she's drinking more soda and less milk than you realized. Does your child bear a resemblance to any of these children?

Billy Butter loves the taste of butter and puts it on everything. He's been known to lick the butter off a slice of bread and then spread more on before eating the bread. He also likes creamy, buttery sauces on vegetables and pasta.

Dairy Donna could live on dairy products. She's particularly partial to milkshakes, cheese, and ice cream.

Lunchmeat Larry won't consider anything for lunch except ham, bologna, salami, or hot dogs.

Sweet Sue doesn't just have one sweet tooth, she has a dozen. She adds sugar to everything and most of her high-fat foods are sweets: cookies, cakes, ice cream, and candy.

Crunchy Charlie goes for high-fat snacks that crunch, especially trail mix and chips. He likes to wash them down with soda—adding a lot of extra calories.

Strategies for Change

There are four basic ways to reduce the amount of excess calories in your child's diet:

- Have high-fat foods less often.
- Have high-fat foods in smaller amounts.
- Have lower-fat items to substitute for high-fat ones.
- Have high-sugar foods less often.

Used in combination, and tailored to your child's food preferences and eating style, these are powerful calorie-lowering strategies. In this chapter, we're going to focus primarily on lower-fat substitutes. In the next two chapters, we'll explore the other three strategies in more detail.

There are three major points to remember as you begin to plan changes:

Make changes gradually. Don't try to abruptly switch your family from red meat every night to fish for dinner five nights in a row.

Make one difficult change at a time. Don't try to switch to reduced-fat salad dressing at the same time you're changing from whole milk to 2%. Even one change a week is good enough.

Make the Pyramid fit your child. Do the best you can and don't panic if he's not yet getting the recommended number of servings from each food group each day or if he eats too many from the tip of the Pyramid. Just keep working gradually toward your goal to improve your child's nutrition while lowering the calories.

Learn About Labels

In the last chapter, we looked at healthy choices on every level of the Pyramid. The charts we provided will point you in the right direction when it comes to substituting lower-fat items for high-fat foods. But, in many cases, we couldn't provide all the details you need because there are so many different products on your store shelves. For example, in the cracker section there are zero-fat varieties, low-fat types, medium-fat choices, and familiar high-fat brands. The only way to distinguish among them is to read the labels. This is true of many different categories of foods. So first we're going to teach you the basics of label reading and then we're going to tour the supermarket sorting out some of the most misleading labels.

Since 1994, all food packages have been required to display more complete information about the nutrients contained in each serving. The labels include information about calories, fat, saturated fat, carbohydrate, fiber, protein, sugars, sodium, cholesterol, and vitamins and minerals. All of this information is important, but for our purposes, in this chapter we are going to focus mostly on interpreting the information about fat and calories.

Somewhere on the package you'll find the heading "Nutrition Facts." Right under this heading is the serving size on which the nutrient amounts are calculated, as well as the number of servings per container. This is important because you may be assuming that a can of soup is one serving, while the manufacturer considers it to be two servings.

The next line displays the number of calories per serving and the number of calories in an individual serving that come from fat. These are the two numbers you need in order to figure what percent of calories in the food are derived from fat. Remember, in the Big Picture of Fat in chapter 11, we gave you the percent of calories from fat in a wide variety of foods. Here's how you can figure the percent fat of any food that has a Nutrition Facts label.

Simply divide the Calories From Fat (sometimes called Fat Calories) by the total Calories and then multiply that number by 100.

For example, if a serving of cereal has 30 fat calories and 210 total calories, you divide 30 by 210 to get .14, which multiplied by 100 equals 14 percent fat. The calculation for a can of chili with 150 fat calories out of 290 calories per serving is 150 ÷ 290 = .52, multiplied by 100 = 52 percent fat.

If you have trouble figuring percentages in your head, you may want to take a pocket calculator with you when you are scouting for new low-fat products or checking out old standbys.

The next portion of the food label provides a list of percentages, but their meaning may not be what you think. Sometimes referred to simply as %DV, they are the percentages of the Daily Values provided by one serving. The daily values are calculated based on an average intake of 2,000 calories per day and indicate the percent of the daily requirement for the various nutrients one would get by eating a serving of the food in the package. With the chili, for example, the line about fat looks like this:

Amount/Serving	%DV
Total Fat 17g	26%

This may appear as though the chili gets 26 percent of its calories from fat. But we already calculated that it's really 52 percent. So what's the deal? The 26% DV means that for a person who eats 2,000 calories a day, one serving of this chili provides 26 percent of the total amount of fat he or she should consume in an *entire* day.

With this understanding of the %DV, you can use it to spot very high-fat or very low-fat foods. Do you really want one serving of food to provide a quarter of your child's daily fat intake? On the other hand, if the %DV for fat is 5 percent, as it was on the cereal, you can see at a glance that it's a low-fat food. Although your child may eat less (or more) than 2,000 calories a day, the %DV is close enough to use as a guide.

Percent Fat Targets

The overall goal is for your child to get no more than 30 percent of his or her total calories from fat. And while it is not necessary to hit this number every day, if you looked at a week's worth of food, it should balance out to about 30 percent calories from fat.

But we're not suggesting that you calculate every morsel of food your child eats. Instead, you can use the following general guidelines to find low-fat selections from each food group. If you keep the majority of your everyday shopping in these lower-fat ranges, it will allow room to balance with higher-fat treats and favorites.

Food Group	Fat Goal
Vegetables and Fruits	0%
Grains	up to 25%
Dairy	up to 30%
Meats	up to 30%

As always, these goals have to be tempered by reality. Low-fat or fat-free foods that are completely rejected by your child and family aren't worth buying. For example, 2% milk gets 35 percent of its calories from fat, while fat-free milk is 6 percent fat. If you switch to fat-free because it fits into the goal for dairy products, but your child stops drinking milk because she can't stand that "blue milk," try 1% milk. It has 20 percent calories from fat and tastes remarkably like 2%. If your child is very particular, you can try mixing 1% and 2% for a while, to wean down to 1%, or just let her have 2% milk and cut fat somewhere else. But whatever you do, don't jeopardize your child's nutrition in the name of low fat.

Red Flags

In addition to the Nutrition Facts labels required on packaged foods, some manufacturers take it upon themselves to make other claims on their product labels. Terms such as "light," "lean," and "reduced cholesterol" are called "key words" by the food industry, but we refer to them as "red flags." While some red flags can alert you to a possible low-fat product your family would enjoy, others can be misleading.

Here's how the government defines these words, as well as some other things we think you should know.

Key Words	Official Definition	Red Flag
Calorie Free	Fewer than 5 calories per serving	May contain artificial sweetener.
Light (Lite)	$\frac{1}{3}$ fewer calories; or no more than $\frac{1}{2}$ the fat of the higher-calorie, higher-fat version; or no more than $\frac{1}{2}$ the sodium of the higher-sodium version	Note that light/lite can refer to sodium instead of fat. Could still be high in fat, although better than the original.
Fat Free	Less than 0.5 gram of fat per serving	May be high in sugar.
Low Fat	3 grams of fat (or less) per serving	If the product is a processed vegetable, you may not want one with that much fat. Three grams of fat added to a serving of green beans makes them 59% fat.
Reduced or Less Fat	At least 25% less fat per serving than the higher-fat version	If the higher-fat version is 100% fat, you may still be getting 75% fat with the reduced-fat product.
Low in Saturated Fat	1 gram saturated fat (or less) per serving	This product can still have a high total fat content if it contains fats that aren't saturated.
Cholesterol Free	Less than 2 milligrams of cholesterol and 2 grams (or less) of saturated fat per serving	Only animal products contain cholesterol. A food can contain no cholesterol and still be extremely high in fat— oil is an example.
Low Cholesterol	20 milligrams of cholesterol (or less) and 2 grams of saturated fat (or less) per serving	See above.

Key Words	Official Definition	Red Flag
Sugar Free	Less than 0.5 gram of sugar per serving	May contain artificial sweetener. Also, may be high in fat.
High Fiber	5 grams of fiber (or more) per serving	May be high in fat or sugar.
Good Source of Fiber	2.5 to 4.9 grams of fiber per serving	See above.

Supermarket Strategies

Shopping is the first step to getting the right food into your house. You know the computer adage: "Garbage in, garbage out"? Well, it's the same thing with groceries. The better the food is that you bring into your house—in terms of good nutrition and low fat—the better it will be for your chubby child and the entire family.

We're going to take you on a tour of the supermarket, stopping at strategic points along the way. Since we can't detail every aisle and every section, we've chosen the ones where the labels are most likely to be confusing or reveal surprising information.

When you go shopping, a good strategy might be to take ten minutes each time to explore one section. Start in the area that contains the largest number of the high-fat or high-sugar foods you circled on your child's Food Records. You may be surprised at the variety and range of fat in such sections as crackers, cookies, lunchmeats, and cheeses.

Regardless of whether you're just running into the market for one meal or stocking up for a week or more, you should plan ahead and go with a list. And for a while, also go with a plan to explore new low-fat options.

Ground Meat

Ground meat is a favorite of many children and it's convenient for the cook because it can be made into so many different dishes. Although we've given you tips for reducing the fat when you cook ground meat, it's even better to start off with varieties that are naturally lower in fat.

The labels on ground beef are particularly confusing because they often have percentages that relate to the fat content. What you need to know is that these numbers do *not* indicate the percent of calories from fat—they refer to the percent of the ground beef's *weight* that comes from fat, which is not the same thing at all. Although every package of meat is different, in general here's how it works:

What the Package Says	Percent Calories From Fat Could Be
Not to exceed 30% fat by weight	50–55%
Not to exceed 22% fat by weight	40–50%
Not to exceed 18% fat by weight	35–40%
Not to exceed 12% fat by weight	30–35%

Your best bet is to pick the leanest your butcher has to offer. If you want to get even leaner, consider mixing ground turkey with the ground beef. But you'll want to use ground turkey breast, sometimes labeled "extra lean," because it has just 12 percent calories from fat. Ground turkey simply labeled "lean" contains dark meat and skin, which hikes the fat to 44 percent—no better than most ground beef. Mixing ground turkey breast with ground beef works well in dishes like meatloaf, spaghetti sauce, tacos, and burritos. You may even want to try using ground turkey breast by itself in some recipes, such as spaghetti sauce, if your family adapts well to the half-and-half.

We would also like to say a word about ground chicken. The package we picked up in the supermarket had 180 calories per serving with 100 *fat* calories, for a whopping 56 percent calories from fat. So beware. Chicken may be low-fat, but packaged ground chicken probably isn't.

Lunchmeat and Hot Dogs

Hot dogs and kids just seem to go together. But, at up to 85 percent fat for regular hot dogs, you may want to check out some of the lower-fat brands. Some are as low as 21 percent fat. And with his favorite condiments (pickles, mustard, ketchup), your child may like one of these brands just as well as the sky-high-fat dogs.

There are lots of low-fat and even nonfat varieties of sliced ham, turkey, chicken, etc. But if your child is a salami fan, the leanest we found was "light" salami with 5 grams less fat per serving than regular. It's still 64 percent fat, but that's somewhat better than 75 percent for the regular kind. The light variety also had significantly fewer calories per serving than the regular salami—70 compared to 120 calories. One strategy you could use here is to balance two slices of light salami in a sandwich for the flavor your child loves, along with low-fat turkey for the nutrition he needs.

Cheese

In the cheese section, when you're drawn to the red flags: "Less Fat" and "Light," pick up the package and figure the percent fat. Most reduced-fat cheeses average 50 percent of calories from fat. But, compared to 65 to 90 percent for regular cheeses, this is a real improvement in a high-nutrition food that most children love. When scanning the cheese section, look for varieties with 6 grams of fat or less per ounce. Yes, there are fat-free cheeses, and if your family likes them, great! But as always, don't sacrifice taste and risk losing out on good nutrition.

Butter and Margarine

Butter is 100 percent fat, as is regular margarine. However, there are a variety of lower-fat and fat-free margarines available. The labels on the lower-fat margarines can be confusing because you'll find that these spreads are 100 percent fat, just like their higher-fat counterparts. The difference is that some of the fat has been replaced with water, which has no calories. So the result is fewer calories and fewer fat calories per teaspoon in the lower-fat varieties, but they're still all fat. With fat-free margarine, you get what its label says—no fat. Although these margarines may be acceptable for spreads, because of their high water content they may not work in cooking. But you can give them a try—they may work in some recipes.

Cereals

Except for some regular granolas, there's not much fat in the cereal aisle. The important thing to be aware of in this section is the large amount of added sugar. On the label, sugar is listed in grams and every 4 grams equals a teaspoon of sugar.

Many traditional kids' cereals are excessively high in sugar, but some are surprisingly low. For example, Kix has just 3 grams of sugar and Cheerios contains just 1 gram of sugar per serving. Compare these to some cereals with as much as 20 grams of sugar per serving—that's equal to five teaspoons of sugar. It's better to buy a low-sugar cereal and let your child add a teaspoon at the table; or better yet, top the cereal with fruit to provide the extra sweetness. It's a good way to get a serving of fruit, too.

If your child is in love with a particular high-sugar cereal, maybe you could find a compatible low-sugar one to mix with it to dilute the total sugar content of her breakfast.

Soups

The soup section is full of choices that are high in nutrition and low in fat. Also, many vegetables that children won't eat "plain" may be perfectly acceptable in soup. Lentil, split pea, and black bean soups are excellent sources of protein and fiber and are usually quite low in fat. The ones we found at the market ranged from 10 to 20 percent calories from fat. Best of all, most children love soup. It's warm, comforting, and filling for an empty little stomach.

In this section you really have to read the Nutrition Facts, because the labels on the front of the soup cans can be deceptive. In general, creamy soups, such as clam chowder, are high in fat. One can we picked up got 50 percent of its calories from fat. But a low-fat clam chowder next to it was just 27 percent fat. Bean with bacon soup sounds as though it would be high in fat because of the bacon; but the ones we saw were about 20 percent fat because they really don't contain very much bacon. On the other hand, the innocent-sounding chicken corn chowder (chicken and corn are both low-fat, right?) had a surprising 56 percent calories from fat.

Salad Dressings

Salad dressing has to taste good or your child won't eat the salad, defeating the whole point. Many children prefer raw vegetables to cooked, so salads are an easy way to get them to eat a serving or two of vegetables. Regular salad dressings are 90 to 100 percent fat, but you can find salad dressing at every percent fat, including zero. Our advice in this section is to choose the lowest-fat dressing that your family truly enjoys. This may involve mixing and matching and a lot of trial and error. But the effort will be worth it if it makes eating salad a pleasure for your child.

If you can't budge the family from high-fat dressing, try using less of it or dilute the fat by adding extra vinegar and water. If they like Thousand Island, you can make it with reduced-fat mayonnaise.

Rice and Noodles

Plain rice and noodles contain no fat, but rice and noodle mixes are another story. We found the labels on these products particularly tricky because some give the values just for the noodles and the mix, without including the margarine or butter called for in the instructions. Most give values both ways, so look for the column with the heading "as prepared" for more accurate figures. The good news: Some mixes contain directions for lower-fat preparation options. Or you can just follow the regular instructions, but use half or none of the fat.

Cookies, Crackers, and Chips

Cookies and crackers can go from 0 to 50 when it comes to percent fat. If your child is old enough, she may be interested in reading the labels and picking out lower-fat crackers herself. Beware of the combination cheese and cracker packs. They're loaded with fat. A lower-fat alternative is to give your child a few low-fat crackers and an individual package of string cheese. It's also a lot less expensive than the prepackaged varieties.

When it comes to cookies, fat is an important consideration, but don't forget about sugar. Sugar can make even fat-free cookies "fattening." For example, an Oreo cookie has 50 calories, with 18 coming from fat, while a fat-free Snackwell Devil's Food cookie has the same 50 calories with 0 fat.

Regular potato chips are 60 to 70 percent fat. There are reduced-fat varieties that are around 45 percent fat. That's still high, but it's better. Also on the market are baked potato chips. Will your family go for chips without fat? Why not give them a try and see?

Other Snacks and Treats

Toaster pastries may seem like breakfast foods, but they're really not. Although there are a number of low-fat flavors, they're really more like a piece of low-fat pie than a nutritious start to the day. Because of their empty calories, they are best used as treats.

Be aware that fruit roll-ups and chewy fruit snacks do not have the same good nutrition as dried fruit. With 100 calories (all from sugar), they're more like candy. However, put into perspective, they are a lower-fat, lower-calorie treat than a 250-calorie candy bar that's 50 percent fat. Fruit rolls could be good substitutes for those big boxes of candy at the movies.

Hot cocoa mix made with water is a low-fat, sweet treat. The ones we looked at were less than 10 percent fat. But you can increase the nutrition a lot and the fat just a little if you make the mix with 1% or nonfat milk instead of water.

Do you have a family of chocoholics? If so, you may want to treat them occasionally to a batch of brownies. Choose a low-fat mix for just 15 percent fat, compared to regular brownies at 40 percent fat and up. The only problem is that the mix makes a large pan, so unless you have a big family, you may want to share some of the brownies with your neighbor.

Peanut Butter

Peanut butter is a staple of many children's lunches. Although it's about 74 percent fat, it provides excellent nutrition. And maybe your child will go for a reduced-fat variety. We found one that was 58 percent fat. Also, if you put jelly or sliced bananas in the sandwich, you can use less peanut butter.

Frozen Foods

In the freezer compartment, you'll find a wide array of frozen desserts, from ice cream to frozen yogurt to juice bars. Frozen yogurt and low-fat ice cream have less fat than regular ice cream, but there is great variety among these frozen desserts. Some are truly low-fat, while others are closer than you may think to the fat and calorie content of some ice creams. Look for frozen yogurt or low-fat ice cream with 4 grams or less of fat per serving.

And also be on the lookout for total calories per serving—even fat-free frozen desserts are usually high in sugar. Choose the lowest-calorie variety that your family enjoys.

There are too many different frozen foods and packaged dinners to detail here. But we would like to make a point about frozen vegetables. In general, try to use the ones that are prepared without fat. But if your child needs his vegetables dressed up, look for some reduced-fat vegetable dishes. We saw a reduced-fat creamed spinach that was only 30 percent fat. However, many of the sauced frozen vegetables were closer to 45 percent fat, so keep reading those labels.

In chapter 15, we'll help you with strategies for making gradual, incremental changes and for helping your child eat high-fat and high-sugar items less often or in smaller quantities. We'll also show you how to put together all of the new information you've learned to plan low-fat, nutritious meals that your child will really like.

15

Calorie-Lowering Strategies Especially for Kids

WHAT DO YOU THINK your child would put in the shopping cart if given the opportunity to go through the supermarket and pick his or her four favorite foods? A dietitian writing for our local paper let seven boys and girls between the ages of seven and nine do just that. Guess what they chose? High-calorie items—cookies, ice cream, chocolate candy, doughnuts, and barbecue potato chips—filled most of the baskets. Other often-selected favorites were low-fat, sugary foods, such as high-sugar cereal and fruit punch. Watermelon, apple-sauce, fruit-flavored yogurt, and canned tuna were the only favorites that were low in fat and provided good nutrition.

When asked to go back through the aisles for their four favorite *nutritious* foods, the baskets got quite a bit lighter. Well represented were fruits, including not only watermelon, but apples, bananas, strawberries, and pineapple. Yogurt was picked by several of the children, as was cheese and low-fat or fat-free milk. The only vegetable chosen was creamed corn. Some high-sugar, low-fat items made it into their "nutritious" baskets—including fruit punch and Jell-O.

What are your child's favorite foods, the items she asks you to get when you go to the market, or requests for a special-occasion dinner? You may already know what they are, but if you are sharing this book with your child, this would be a good opportunity to ask her what her very favorite foods are. You can record them here, along with the Fat/Nutrition Rating of each:

- *Low Fat/High Nutrition* ($\downarrow$F $\uparrow$N): any food in the low-fat cate-gories in each of the Pyramid's food groups, except for those marked with an asterisk, which means they are high in sugar. Those low-fat, high-sugar foods such as animal crackers and frozen yogurt belong in the low-fat/low-nutrition category below because the majority of their calories come from sugar.
- *High Fat/High Nutrition* ($\uparrow$F $\uparrow$N): high-fat foods that contain substantial amounts of protein, calcium, and other nutrients, such as iron. These foods might include meats and cheeses and other high-fat dairy products.
- *High Fat/Low Nutrition* ($\uparrow$F $\downarrow$N): high-fat food in the tip of the Pyramid, as well as some high-fat, high-sugar choices in the Bread and Milk groups, such as pastries and ice cream.
- *Low Fat/Low Nutrition* ($\downarrow$F $\downarrow$N): mostly low-fat/high-sugar items, such as sodas, juice drinks, low-fat cookies, and sugar-type candy.

Here are two examples, using the items chosen by two of the children in the newspaper article:

Food	Fat/Nutrition Rating
Watermelon	$\downarrow$F $\uparrow$N
Low-fat yogurt	$\downarrow$F $\uparrow$N
Tuna (water pack)	$\downarrow$F $\uparrow$N
Chocolate chip ice cream	$\uparrow$F $\downarrow$N

Food	Fat/Nutrition Rating
Chocolate ice cream	$\uparrow$F $\downarrow$N
Doughnuts	$\uparrow$F $\downarrow$N
Cookies	$\uparrow$F $\downarrow$N
Fruit punch	$\downarrow$F $\downarrow$N

Now fill in the blanks for your child:

Food	Fat/Nutrition Rating
_____	_____
_____	_____
_____	_____
_____	_____
_____	_____
_____	_____

You're ahead of the game if your child has one or two favorites that fall in the low-fat/high-nutrition category. Perhaps he truly loves some fruits, vegetables, grains, low-fat dairy products, and meats. If so, be sure to serve them *often*.

The overall strategy for favorite foods in the other categories is "moderation." Remember, there's no such thing as a bad food. But you can work toward serving low-nutrition or high-fat foods (1) less often, (2) in smaller quantities, or (3) less often and in smaller quantities. This way, your child still gets to enjoy her very favorite foods—but maybe not every day.

Of course, "less often" and "in smaller quantities" are relative terms. They are based on how often and how much your child currently eats a particular food. For example, if your child is used to having a rich dessert with lunch and dinner every day, less often might mean cutting down to dessert only once a day—either at lunch or dinner. Or if he's currently eating his favorite food, potato chips, once a day, you might try cutting down to every other day. Small children, especially, can deal better with, "No cupcake today, but you can have one tomorrow," than having to wait until "next week," which seems an eternity away.

The smaller quantity approach could be applied to a youngster who is accustomed to having four to five cookies and a soda as an afternoon snack. Try cutting down to two to three cookies, and substitute a glass of low-fat milk for the soda; then cut down to one to two cookies, the milk, and maybe a small piece of fruit to make up the difference. Or a smaller quantity might mean serving a small scoop of ice cream for dessert, instead of filling the bowl to the brim.

In addition to generally trying to reduce the amount of high-fat or low-nutrition foods your child eats, here are some strategies specific to each of the categories.

High Fat/High Nutrition

This is the good news/bad news category. On the one hand, these foods are definitely high in fat, but on the other, they provide your child with the good nutrition she needs to grow. So you may want to let her eat these favorites more frequently, but balance them with lower-fat foods. Or you may be able to find ways to reduce the fat, while keeping the nutrition and taste. Here are some examples:

- *Peanut butter:* See if she likes a reduced-fat variety.
- *Grilled cheese sandwiches:* Instead of grilling the sandwich in butter, try toasting the bread. Then top one slice with the cheese and melt it in the oven or toaster oven before putting the other piece of toast on top.
- *Pizza:* Try to limit the high-fat toppings, such as sausage and pepperoni, while adding a few vegetables for color and flavor.

High Fat/Low Nutrition

Your child deserves to enjoy his favorites from this category, too—but not all the time. One way to cut down is to try some lower-fat substitutions. But be aware that while the replacements are lower in fat, most are also quite low in nutrition and high in sugar and should be eaten in moderation, too.

- *Ice cream:* Find out if frozen yogurt or low-fat ice cream would satisfy her taste for the real thing.
- *Chocolate:* Take advantage of all the low-fat and fat-free chocolate cookies, cakes, and cupcakes on the market. But watch the portion size because fat-free isn't *calorie*-free. To boost the nutrition of these chocolate treats, serve them with a glass of low-fat or fat-free milk. A cup of chocolate low-fat milk or hot cocoa

made with fat-free milk is another nutritious way to satisfy a chocolate craving.

- *Cookies:* Is it a specific brand that she loves? If so, maybe there's a lower-fat version of her favorite cookie right there next to it on the store shelf. If she's not picky and loves all kinds of cookies, experiment and see if she would enjoy some of the fat-free varieties. And if her favorite is a homemade cookie, see if you can modify the recipe to cut down on the fat and sugar, but only if it doesn't alter the taste or texture enough to demote the cookie from "favorite" to "just okay."
- *Chips:* If your child likes snacks that crunch, he may not object to crunching on low-fat snacks instead of high-fat ones. Try pretzels, popcorn, and low-fat trail mix you can make with pretzels, dry cereal, and dried fruit. Or if nothing can substitute for chips, try a lower-fat or fat-free variety. If he doesn't like fat-free chips by themselves, maybe they would be more acceptable if you serve them with a dip that just happens to be low-fat, such as salsa, fat-free bean dip, or a creamy dip made with yogurt or fat-free sour cream.

Low Fat/Low Nutrition

The most likely favorites in this category are sodas and juice drinks. Both should be allowed in moderation. One way to cut down on soda consumption is to avoid buying big bottles. Volume is easier to control with individual cans, perhaps limiting your child to one per day. Try to get her into the habit of drinking water when she's thirsty instead of always quenching her thirst with a sweet drink.

Many high-fat or low-nutrition foods your child eats might not ever make it onto his "favorites" list. So, we have a variety of fat-lowering strategies for some of these everyday foods, all in keeping with our theme of making gradual, incremental changes that your child and your family can live with.

Added Fats

As we have seen, low-fat foods can be quickly turned into high-fat ones with the addition of pure fat toppings: butter, margarine, mayonnaise, and oil. And while it's easy to say, "Just leave them off," it's not so easy to do. Instead, we suggest you gradually work toward less added fat. And then see if you can make it "no fat" some of the time.

Like Butter Billy, your child may have a particular love for some pure fats. But consider whether quantity is more important to him than the type of butter, margarine, or mayonnaise. Some children don't care if the margarine is reduced-calorie or even fat-free, as long as they get plenty of it on their baked potatoes. Likewise, some children will accept lower-fat mayonnaise as long as you don't skimp on it when making a sandwich.

Other children want "the real thing"—but are willing to have less of it. Perhaps your child would be happier with a little real butter on her baked potato and none on her bread, rather than a low-fat sub-stitute she dislikes on both. In the same way, some children would rather have mustard on their sandwich than "phony mayonnaise," or would be happier with a mixture of mustard and real mayonnaise than something imitation.

Don't forget the other pure fat—oil. While the bottle of oil doesn't usually make it to the dinner table (unless, perhaps, you're dipping your bread into olive oil), oil often is added during the cooking of fresh food. You can cut down on oil by using less of it in recipes, sub-stituting vegetable cooking spray to keep foods from sticking, and using reduced-fat margarine or broth instead of oil to cook some foods.

Mixing

Mixing a high-fat food with its lower-fat counterpart is a strategy that can be used by itself or as part of a gradual process to switch com-pletely to the lower-fat item. Try mixing:

- regular mayonnaise with reduced-fat or fat-free mayonnaise
- regular or reduced-fat mayonnaise with mustard
- reduced-fat mayonnaise with fat-free plain yogurt
- whole milk with 2% milk
- 2% milk with 1% milk
- 1% milk with fat-free milk
- regular salad dressing with reduced-fat or fat-free dressing
- 1 whole egg with 1 or 2 egg whites
- lean or leanest ground beef with ground turkey breast

Increasing Fruits and Vegetables

Another calorie-lowering strategy involves increasing the amount of vegetables and fruits your child eats. Not only is this good from a nutrition standpoint, but filling up on these naturally low-fat foods leaves less room for high-fat items. The challenge is to find ways to get your child to enjoy more of these low-fat, nutritious foods.

Most children like fruit, so perhaps all you have to do is make a variety more accessible to your child. And adding a little fun to fruit will add to its popularity. Here are some ideas:

- Wash the grapes, cut them into little bunches, and put them at kid-level in the refrigerator. Or try freezing them for a cool treat.
- Peel and section oranges or cut them in quarters with the peel on to make them easier to eat.
- Cut apples into four to eight slices for easy munching.
- Try our recipe on page 283 for frozen bananas.
- Top sliced fresh fruit, such as strawberries or peaches, with a little low-fat yogurt. Or put cut-up fruit with a little juice in the blender for a fruit smoothie.
- Take your child on an outing to a fruit farm where he can pick his own strawberries, cherries, peaches, apricots, or other really fresh fruit.

Increasing vegetable consumption can be a little more challenging, but these strategies may help:

- Be a role model—how can you expect your child to eat spinach or broccoli if you can't eat them without making a face?
- When you're shopping, let your child decide which vegetables to buy.
- Let your youngster help when you prepare or cook the vegetables. Little hands can shell peas, peel carrots, or husk corn. When children fix something themselves, they tend to want to like it.
- Buy kid-sized vegetables, such as baby corn, peeled baby carrots, baby zucchini, and little new potatoes.
- Present vegetables in a creative way, such as putting a variety of small or cut-up vegetables on kebabs on the grill when you barbecue.

- Try low-fat sauces to put over hot vegetables or low-fat dips for children to dunk raw vegetables in. Try a variety of crunchy dunkers, such as baby carrots, celery sticks, red bell pepper strips, jicama slices, and broccoli trees.
- Don't force or bribe your child to eat vegetables. Children know instinctively that if the vegetables were really good you wouldn't be bribing them to eat them. You don't force them to eat chocolate cake, do you?
- Keep trying. Children's tastes change as they get older. They also tend to like what they become familiar with. Research shows that it may take up to ten tries (spaced out over a period of time) before your child learns to like a particular vegetable.

Non-favorite Foods

We've saved the easiest category for last: high-fat foods that your child isn't particularly fond of. Most you can eliminate easily. They won't even be missed. Maybe she isn't crazy about mayonnaise but needs something to moisten her sandwiches. Try mustard, ketchup, or fat-free margarine. Perhaps she wouldn't mind having jam or jelly on her bagel instead of butter or margarine. Use the charts in chapter 13 for more low-fat ideas.

Putting It All Together

We've given you a lot of food for thought in the last three chapters. Your job is to take the information and begin making gradual changes that will help your overweight child.

To help you see how it might work, we have put together a week's worth of meals and snacks that illustrate twenty-three of the specific strategies we have shared with you (see page 150). This is *not* a recommended meal plan for you to follow: it's just an example of how the strategies might be applied. We have also chosen this combination of meals and snacks to demonstrate the flexible application, over the course of a week, of the following basic nutrition goals:

- Eat a variety of foods.
- Eat the recommended number of servings from each Food Group.
- Have 30 percent or fewer calories from fat.

The key word is flexible. You will notice, for example, that Saturday and Sunday don't include five servings of vegetables and fruits, and that some days don't have six servings of grains. Also, if you did a lot of calculations, you would see that each meal doesn't work out to 30 percent calories from fat; neither does every day. However, it averages out to about 30 percent calories from fat for the whole week because we applied a mixture of our three overall fat-lowering strategies:

- Have high-fat foods less often.
- Have high-fat foods in smaller portions.
- Have lower-fat choices to substitute for high-fat foods.

The numbers we've given to the specific strategies below refer to selected items in the Week's Worth of Meals and Snacks that demonstrate how the strategy might be applied:

1. When you serve juice, try to make it high in vitamin C.
2. Serve whole grains.
3. Don't go too low-fat if it would compromise good nutrition. It doesn't have to be fat-free milk.
4. Shop low-fat.
5. There are no bad foods—include high-fat or high-sugar treats sparingly during the week.
6. Pretzels or light microwave popcorn are good crunchy substitutes for chips.
7. Use reduced-fat salad dressing when you can—it doesn't have to be fat-free.
8. Choose the leanest ground beef.
9. Use reduced-fat margarine and mayonnaise when the taste is acceptable.
10. Keep high-fat nutritious foods, like peanut butter, but balance them with low-fat foods.
11. Make fruits and vegetables appealing.
12. Soup is a good place to get a serving of vegetables.
13. Use low-fat cooking techniques—oven-baking "fries" instead of frying, for example.
14. Have high-fat favorites in smaller quantities.
15. Use ground turkey breast in recipes instead of ground beef.
16. Choose vegetables that are good sources of Vitamin A.

Example of a Week's Worth of Meals

Day	Breakfast	Snack	Lunch
Mon.	• Orange juice[1] • Oatmeal[2] • 1% milk[3]	• Banana	• Water-pack tuna[4] with reduced-fat mayo, lettuce, and tomato in a pita pocket • Small bag of chips[5] • Quartered apple • 2% milk (from cafeteria)
Tues.	• Orange slices • Toaster waffle with reduced-fat margarine[9] and syrup • 1% milk	• Low-fat granola bar	• Peanut butter[10] and jelly sandwich on whole wheat bread[2] • Celery sticks • 2% milk
Wed.	• Dry cereal topped with sliced banana and 1% milk • 1% milk (to drink)	• Baggie of pretzels	• Sandwich with 2 slices of turkey breast, 2 slices of Italian salami[14] on rye bread with mustard • Quartered orange • 2% milk
Thurs.	• Pineapple juice • Toast with melted part-skim mozzarella cheese	• Baby raw carrots[16]	• Fruit yogurt • Banana • Whole wheat bread with low-fat margarine • 2 low-fat cookies[17]
Fri.	• Cranberry[1]-grape juice • Toasted English muffin with low-fat margarine and jelly	• Box of raisins	• Low-fat ham and cheese sandwich on rye bread with mustard[19] and lettuce • Sliced cucumbers • 2% milk
Sat.	• Orange juice • Scrambled egg—1 egg plus 1 egg white[21] • Toast with jam	• Melon balls[11]	• Fast-food hamburger • Small French fries[5] • 2% milk
Sun.	• Homemade pancakes with maple syrup[22] • 2 link sausages • 1% milk	• Fresh pear	• Bagel and light cream cheese • 1% milk • Baby raw carrots

and Snacks for a Ten-Year-Old Child

Snack	Dinner	Snack
• Baggie of pretzels[6]	• Salad with reduced-fat dressing[7] • Meatloaf—leanest ground beef[8] • Mashed potatoes • Green beans • 1% milk	• Low-fat frozen yogurt[20]
• Strawberries topped with fruit yogurt[11]	• Vegetable soup[12] • Baked chicken leg • Oven French "fries"[13] • Fresh zucchini • 1% milk	• Homemade low-fat muffin[13] • Apple juice
• Microwave light popcorn[6]	• Salad with reduced-fat dressing • Spaghetti and sauce made with ground turkey breast[15] • French bread • 1% milk	• Watermelon • 10 animal crackers[17]
• Ice cream cone[5]	• Soft chicken taco with beans, low-fat cheese, lettuce, and tomato[18] • Rice cooked in broth • 1% milk	• Homemade orange juice bar
• Baked apple topped with frozen yogurt[20]	• Homemade pizza with fresh vegetables and shredded low-fat cheese[18] • Salad with reduced-fat dressing • 1% milk	• Candy bar[5] • 1% milk
• Baked potato chips • 12-ounce can of soda[24]	• Low-fat macaroni and cheese[18] • Salad • 1% milk	• Frozen yogurt[20] • Low-fat cookie[17]
• Low-fat granola bar	• Sloppy Chicken Joe's • Cut-up raw vegetables • 1% milk	• Hot cocoa made with 1% milk[23]

17. Substitute low-fat for high-fat varieties of cookies and crackers, but keep your eye on quantity.
18. Pare down the fat in high-fat, high-nutrition foods.
19. Substitute mustard for mayonnaise.
20. Substitute frozen yogurt for ice cream.
21. Mixing helps lower the fat.
22. Don't add pure fats if they're not necessary—butter may not be needed with syrup.
23. Hot cocoa can be a chocolate substitute.
24. Limit volume of soda and other sugary drinks.

Keep in mind that we are not suggesting you use all of the strategies given in the chart, at least not right away. Start by picking a few that address some of your child's high-fat habits. Then try a few more as you figure out which ones work and which ones don't. In time, you'll have your own repertoire of calorie-lowering strategies tailored to your child and your entire family.

16

Meals and Snacks: How Much, How Often?

TOO MUCH OF A GOOD THING—whether it's sunshine or food—is still too much. And just as we can be fooled into thinking that our children won't get sunburned on an overcast day, we can mistakenly believe that if they eat low-fat food, they won't get fat.

Children put on excess weight because the number of calories they consume is greater than the amount they use in their daily activities. The fat-lowering and sugar-lowering strategies we've given you so far will go a long way toward reducing both fat calories and total calories in your child's diet. But calories, even low-fat ones, can add up if a youngster eats too much.

The amount of food a child eats is a delicate issue. Remember, our Child's Bill of Rights says, "Children have the right to eat as much or as little as they need." But if your child is consistently eating more than she needs, you have the responsibility to help her learn how much is enough.

In our Eating Behavior Survey on page 30, you identified a number of reasons your child might reach for food. All of the reasons you identified, including being truly hungry, can lead to *over*-eating. In this chapter, we will offer you a variety of different strategies to address the particular reason or reasons your child may be eating too much or too often.

Eating for Reasons Other Than Hunger

Children, like adults, sometimes eat because they are bored, tired, stressed, angry, upset, or sad. Try to help your child deal with these emotions in ways that are more effective than by eating.

If he's bored and has nothing to do besides make trips to the refrigerator, offer to do something fun with him—play a game or work on a project together. If you're too busy, help him find something to do alone or suggest that he invite a friend over to play. If boredom is a recurrent issue, you may need to help him identify some regular activities to fill up his schedule.

When your child is tired, a cookie may taste good, but it won't perk her up as much as a nap or a walk around the block. If she's eating because she's stressed, angry, upset, or sad, the food might make her feel better temporarily. But talking about the reasons for her distress will be more effective in the long run, especially if gaining weight is causing her stress.

Another reason for eating when not hungry is procrastination. Grabbing a snack is a great excuse for delaying homework or temporarily suspending some other disagreeable task. If your child just needs a break, encourage him to call a friend on the phone, play a quick video game, or walk the dog.

Nonhunger eating also occurs when food is used as a reward. If you currently offer food rewards to your child for good behavior, good grades, or doing extra chores, try to think of other ways to recognize her efforts. Perhaps a trip to the park or the beach, reading her a story, or letting her pick out a toy, game, or CD would send a better message than rewarding her with food.

Eating by Association

Does your child tend to associate certain activities with food? Does he have to have popcorn at the movies, chips and dip while watching television, or a bowl of ice cream to make homework more palatable? Chances are these are family patterns that your child has learned. These kinds of habits are difficult to change, so you might first try limiting the *amount* of food eaten on such occasions. For example, at the movies, buy a smaller box of popcorn for the whole family to share.

As for snacking while watching TV, if the viewers usually grab whatever they crave at the moment, try to provide a more defined snack that they choose in advance. And make it clear that they do not get a new snack with each TV program. Also, it helps to serve low-fat, low-calorie TV snacks, such as raw vegetables or air-popped popcorn.

And if food makes the homework go down better, let her eat her afternoon snack while doing it. Or if she does her schoolwork after dinner, maybe she will see the merit of saving her dessert to help her get through her assignments.

Eating When Others Eat

Some children eat because their friends or siblings are eating and they want to be part of the group. If your child is trying to slim down, try to discuss the issue of extra calories with him. Point out that since his main goal is to participate in the social activity, he could share a smaller helping of the food and a larger helping of the fun.

A child's desire to eat also may be triggered by seeing others eating food that looks particularly appetizing. In this instance, you can help by not having his most-tempting foods in the house too often—unless they're low-fat and low-calorie.

Eating Continuously

Some children are in the habit of eating all the time; as soon as they finish a meal, they're back in the kitchen looking for a snack. This is where one of your parental responsibilities from chapter 10 comes in: to emphasize mealtimes and provide appropriate snacks. As we've said, a child should have three predictable meals, plus two to three snacks, a day. If your child is able to count on eating five to six times during the day, she probably won't need to eat more. Predictability is key. If she knows she will be able to eat soon, it's easier to wait. It is also important to provide snacks and meals that pack enough staying power to keep your child from getting hungry again right away. We will explain more about how to do this in the next section.

If your child tends to eat all the time because food is always accessible, it's up to you to make it less readily available. If seeing the food is a trigger for your child's wanting to eat, you can put tempting snacks in hard-to-find places. Keeping children occupied and away from the kitchen can also be an effective strategy. Especially with younger children, distraction can work wonders. If your child is older and trying to control her weight, you may be able to brainstorm ideas with her for alternate activities when she has the urge to eat, but isn't really hungry.

Being Too Hungry

Coming to the table too hungry is one of the most common reasons that children, and adults, overeat at meals. When we're ravenous, we want to eat until that gnawing feeling goes away. The problem is that our stomachs are satisfied about twenty minutes before our brains get the message. And in those twenty minutes, your child can eat much more than he needs. Eating more slowly can help with this type of overeating problem, but an even better approach is to prevent the "over-hungry" syndrome.

Being too hungry at meals is the result of two factors: going too long without eating or not eating properly at the previous meal or snack.

The obvious solution to over-hunger caused by waiting too long before eating is to add a snack to break up extended periods between meals. If your child eats lunch at noon and supper isn't served until 7 P.M., that's too long. An appropriate snack after school can help prevent excessive hunger and overeating at dinner.

When planning meals and snacks for your child, it's important to consider not only quantity and timing, but also "staying power." Some foods stay with us longer, while others leave us hungry again in an hour. If you eat an apple, for example, you will get hungrier faster than if you eat a piece of cheese. The reason is that carbohydrate, protein, and fat are digested by our bodies at different rates, and the faster we digest a particular food, the quicker we feel empty again.

Carbohydrates (fruits, vegetables, grains, and sweets) are digested the fastest. Sugars can be absorbed in fifteen to thirty minutes. Fruits and vegetables are digested in thirty minutes to three hours: The more fiber they contain, the longer it takes. Starches may seem filling, but they require just one to three hours to digest—with whole grains taking the longer time, because of their extra fiber content.

Proteins (meat, dairy products, and dried beans) take longer to digest than carbohydrates do because they have a more complex molecular structure. Proteins require two to four hours for digestion.

Fat stays with you twice as long as protein or carbohydrate, but unfortunately provides double the calories. It takes five to seven hours to fully digest high-fat foods.

One of the effects of reducing the amount of fat your child eats is that she may feel hungry a bit sooner after eating. In the absence of excess fat, you have to rely on adequate protein, eaten at strategic times during the day, to keep hunger at bay. Remember, adequate protein is not a lot—just two to three servings a day. Refer to the chart on page 105 for serving sizes by age.

Strategically Placed Protein

Using protein to help control excessive hunger is a matter of timing. A serving of protein usually is part of the evening meal, but it may be completely missing in the ten to twelve waking hours before dinner. Protein at lunch is a logical and easy place for your child to get a second serving. But some children may need a little boost of protein and carbohydrate at other times during the day.

If your child is too hungry and tends to overeat at lunch, here are some strategies you can try. One may solve the problem, or you may have to use several in combination to fit the needs and schedule of your child.

1. Be sure he eats something for breakfast. (We've got lots of flexible ideas in the "Great Way to Start the Day" section later in this chapter.)
2. Add a mid-morning snack. (See the "Smart Snacks" section.)
3. Try adding protein as part of breakfast.
4. If your child eats cereal or toast for breakfast, include some protein, such as a piece of string cheese, as part of the mid-morning snack. (We've included a lot more suggestions in Smart Snacks.)

If your child is too hungry at dinner, the strategies are similar:

1. Be sure she eats a satisfying lunch, with a sufficient amount of protein (approximately 3 ounces) and whole-grain starch.
2. Add a mid-afternoon snack, if she's not getting one.
3. If her normal snack isn't working, make it protein-rich, such as a carton of yogurt or half a tuna sandwich.

Smart Snacks

Snacks have developed a bad reputation. They're usually associated with high-fat, high-calorie treats that provide little or no nutritional value. And while there is a place for occasional treats between meals, when we recommend that you serve two to three snacks a day to your child, we are referring to *smart* snacks. Snacks for children need to be smart because these mini-meals provide a major portion of a child's daily nutrient intake. As much as one-third of a child's daily calories may come from snacks. Smart snacks:

- taste good to your child
- may include some strategically placed protein for staying power
- are timed properly—not too close to a meal
- provide good nutrition
- are low-fat
- are substantial enough to help your child make it to the next meal, but aren't meals in themselves
- are easily accessible to the child if an adult isn't around when the snack is needed
- are planned, so there aren't too many or too few snacks in the day

Here are some suggestions for Smart Snacks your child might enjoy. The ones with significant amounts of protein are marked with a "P."

Crunchy Snacks

- Raw vegetables with reduced-fat dip
- Popcorn, microwave light or air popped
- Pretzels
- Low-fat crackers with reduced-fat cheese[P]
- Trail mix made from dry cereal, pretzels, and dried fruit
- Celery sticks spread thin with peanut butter[P]
- Baked tortilla chips with salsa
- Baked tortilla chips with low-fat bean dip[P]

Savory Snacks

- Vegetable soup
- Lentil or split pea soup[P]

- Chicken noodle soup
- Baked potato topped with cottage cheese[P]
- Fresh fruit and reduced-fat cheese[P]
- Bagel with fat-free cream cheese
- Quesadilla (tortilla with reduced-fat cheese[P] melted on top)
- Half a tuna sandwich[P]
- English muffin topped with pizza sauce and melted low-fat mozzarella cheese[P]
- Carrot-raisin salad with pineapple chunks
- Cottage cheese with fruit[P]
- Green salad with low-fat dressing
- Half a pita with turkey[P], lettuce, and tomato

Sweet Snacks

- Dry cereal and low-fat milk[P]
- Fresh fruit
- Frozen fruit (grapes, melon balls, berries)
- Fruit canned in its own juice
- Applesauce
- Fat-free or low-fat yogurt[P]
- A couple of graham crackers, ginger snaps, or animal crackers with a glass of low-fat milk[P]
- Gelatin with fruit
- Frozen waffle topped with sliced fruit or jam
- Fruit smoothie (frozen fruit, yogurt, and juice)[P]
- Baked apple
- Low-fat muffin
- Snack pack of raisins
- Instant pudding made with fat-free milk
- Fruit juice pops

A Great Way to Start the Day

Skipping breakfast or having just a glass of juice is a setup for overeating at lunch or eating all day to try to satisfy that "empty feeling." Breakfast at home, or at least prepared at home, is more effective for weight control than either breakfast at school or no breakfast at all. When you prepare your child's breakfast, you can influence its content better than if she picks up breakfast on the way to school or buys it in the cafeteria. It is a great opportunity to ensure that she starts her day with a nutritious meal that is low fat, too.

From an educational standpoint, breakfast is the most important meal of the day because it provides a foundation for your youngster to be ready to learn when he gets to school. Studies have shown that children who eat breakfast exhibit better concentration at school, have longer attention spans, and may have better attitudes toward learning than children who start the school day on empty stomachs.

We know that morning schedules are hectic and that breakfast sometimes gets lost in the confusion of getting ready for school and work. Let's take a look at some of the common barriers to children eating breakfast at home and some possible ways to overcome these morning hurdles.

It may be that your child doesn't have time in the morning to sit down and eat. Since it's faster to drink a meal than to eat one, try serving breakfast in a glass. Whip up a breakfast smoothie made from yogurt, fresh fruit, and ice. Or for extra calcium and protein, make the smoothie with fruit yogurt and milk. Another option is to give him something he can eat on the way to school, such as a toasted reduced-fat cheese sandwich or one made with fat-free cold cuts. Or you could spread peanut butter and jelly between two pieces of a toaster waffle— for a waffle sandwich. Any of these breakfast sandwiches would go well with an individual carton of low-fat milk or a box of orange juice.

What if you don't have time in the morning to prepare breakfast for your child? Maybe you can set things up the night before. Put the glass, bowl, spoon, napkin, even the box of cereal on the table. You also could cut up some strawberries or other fruit to go on top of the cereal and have them ready in the refrigerator, along with the milk and juice. This will save you time in the morning or make it easy for your child to finish preparing a healthy, low-fat breakfast for herself.

What if your child isn't hungry for breakfast early in the morning? Try packing her lunchbox with food for breakfast in addition to her lunch. That way she can eat breakfast when she's ready—at recess or between classes. Take another look at the Smart Snack list for portable breakfast ideas.

What if your child doesn't like traditional breakfast food? Who says breakfast has to be cereal or eggs? Try fixing a turkey sandwich on whole wheat bread or a bagel with a smear of peanut butter for breakfast. You can even make a tuna sandwich, with water-pack tuna and reduced-fat mayonnaise.

The Clean-Plate Club and Other Habits

We've spent a lot of time in this chapter focusing on strategies for preventing excessive hunger because it often leads to overeating. But it's not the only reason that children, or adults, overindulge. If you've been trying the strategies we've suggested for curbing excessive hunger and your child still seems to be eating too much at meals, there may be other reasons behind his overeating.

Perhaps he's a member of the Clean-Plate Club. Do you have a rule in your house that children have to finish everything on their plates? Some children get into this habit because cleaning their plates is rewarded with dessert. This is a double whammy when it comes to controlling quantity and managing weight.

You can start reversing this habit by rescinding the Clean-Plate Rule. At the same time you discuss the rule change, you may want to remind all family members to try to serve themselves an amount they think they are hungry enough to finish. But remember, you agreed not to make them eat it all. Be sure that both parents will support this change. It may be especially difficult for the cook to see food go uneaten. It will take time for everyone to adjust, but it's important for your chubby child to learn when he's had enough.

If you don't encourage your child to clean her plate but she's in the habit of doing it anyway, regardless of how much food is on it, what should you do? This is a trickier issue. Ultimately, you would like your child to learn to stop eating when she's satisfied, even if there's some food left on her plate. While you're working slowly toward that goal, you can help her with slightly smaller portions. That way, when she cleans her plate, she will be eating a bit less food. Sometimes you can do this subtly. For example, you can put a little less meat or cheese in her sandwich or buy slightly smaller baking potatoes.

The key to decreasing portion size is to do it slowly, with minimal reductions at any one time. If you serve your child a potato half the size he's used to, he'll notice and perhaps want two to compensate. But if the potato is only 10 to 15 percent smaller, it is more likely to go unnoticed. And when your child serves himself, perhaps you can suggest that he try a smaller *first* helping, but reassure him that he can have seconds if he's still hungry.

Some children eat everything on their plates and immediately ask for seconds. Are second helpings automatic at your dinner table? Rather than *offer* more food, you can wait to see if anyone requests it. Or, you can minimize the temptation for second helpings by keeping the serving dishes off the table—either in the kitchen, if you eat in the dining room, or on the counter or stove, if you eat in the kitchen. Also, if you know your child will want second helpings of food she's particularly fond of, cook only enough for firsts, unless the favorite is low calorie. Another way to reduce quantity and still have second helpings is to encourage smaller servings, both for firsts and seconds.

Another reason children may overeat, whether it's by cleaning their plates or having second helpings or both, is that they need to feel *overly* full in order to be satisfied with a meal. Some children interpret that stuffed feeling as desirable and anything less as still being hungry. This is perhaps the most difficult overeating habit to address. Ideally, we all should learn to stop eating when we are satisfied—no longer hungry, but not stuffed.

One thing you can do is make sure that there are plenty of low-fat, low-calorie foods to round out the meal, such as salad, extra vegetables, and fruits. And with an older child, you might try explaining the difference between satisfied and full and ask her to experiment to see how she feels with a smaller serving. Is she still hungry or does she really feel pretty satisfied? Assure her that if she's hungry, she can have more food. You also might want to tell her about the twenty-minute delay between her stomach being full and her brain getting the message. Then you can suggest that she wait awhile before having second helpings, so she has time to consider whether she's had enough.

Perhaps more than any of the changes we've discussed so far, changes that relate to reducing the volume of food your child eats should be made in small increments and slowly over time. The goal is to help your child develop new habits that will result in his feeling as satisfied eating *less* food as he did when he ate *more*.

17

Eating Away From Home

BREAKFAST IN THE CAR on the way to school, an afternoon snack from a convenience store, dinner at a fast-food restaurant. Does this sound like your child's schedule?

The average American family spends nearly 50 percent of its food budget on meals eaten away from home. One-third of this amount is spent in fast-food restaurants, while the other two-thirds is spent in such locations as traditional restaurants, vending machines, convenience stores, and concession stands.

If your child's diet consists mainly of healthy, nutritious meals and snacks prepared in your own kitchen, you don't have to worry about the occasional restaurant meal or fast-food treat. If, on the other hand, your child eats out as much as he eats in, the food he eats away from home counts a lot more than you may think.

While good nutrition is the goal no matter where the food is eaten, having high-calorie temptations leaping off the menu makes it difficult to make healthful choices in a restaurant. Therefore, compromise, flexibility, and balance are particularly important when eating out with your overweight child. The objective is to try to help your child with choices that are as low fat as possible, in portion sizes appropriate to her needs. But in the process of doing this, it is important not to single out your chubby child for special treatment. A few extra calories or grams of fat are not worth causing her embarrassment or wounding her self-esteem.

Instead, it's best that your whole family try to revise their assumptions about eating away from home. Eating out doesn't have to mean pigging out. We'll show you how to grab a quick bite or enjoy a leisurely meal—without contributing to your child's overweight.

We realize that if your child is older, you're not going to be able to exert much influence on his food choices away from home. However, if he's interested in controlling his weight, he might appreciate the information in this chapter.

Restaurants

What are your considerations when choosing a restaurant for a family breakfast, lunch, or dinner? Most likely you think about such things as cost, type of food, service, and environment when making your decision. How about adding *availability of low-fat choices* to your list? If you pick a restaurant that has lots of healthy menu items, everyone will benefit.

We know that your family, like everyone else's, eats at a variety of different kinds of restaurants. American, Chinese, Italian, and Mexican are likely to be among your family's favorites, so we'll give you strategies for each of these.

But before we get into the specifics, here are a few strategies that can be applied to any restaurant meal:

- Don't go to the restaurant ravenous. It's a setup for overeating, including devouring the basket of bread or tortilla chips, which is put on the table before you even order your meal.
- Role modeling is one of the most effective approaches. When you order low-fat, reasonably sized portions, your child will consider it to be appropriate restaurant behavior.
- As you peruse the menu, casually mention a few of the lower-calorie items you come across. Don't point them out specifically to your child or even mention that the dishes are low fat. It would be more subtle and effective to say: "Hmm. The grilled chicken sounds good." Say it to yourself, but distinctly enough for other family members to hear. Maybe they'll take the hint.
- Restaurant portions tend to be oversized. If you have two young children, perhaps they can share an entree and a salad. Or maybe you can share part of your dinner with your child.

- If there's a high-calorie, family favorite on the menu, try getting one order for the whole table to share. This works particularly well with appetizers and desserts.

American-Style Restaurants

American-style restaurants serve food as varied as our multicultural country, often in casual, child-friendly settings. Their extensive menus generally include a variety of lower-fat items, but we want to make one strong suggestion. Don't make an all-you-can-eat or buffet-style restaurant a regular eating-out destination for your family. This type of food-free-for-all is a setup for your chubby child and the rest of your family. Too many tempting choices in plain view, unrestrained portion sizes, and unlimited servings pose a triple threat to a child working on her weight.

The children's menus at American-style restaurants don't do your child any favors, either. They usually feature such high-fat items as hot dogs, macaroni and cheese, and fried chicken with mashed potatoes.

If you want a smaller portion for your child, why not order an appetizer or even two rather than an appetizer and an entree. However, beware of high-fat starters, such as buffalo chicken wings, fried calamari, nachos, or potato skins. Lower-fat choices might include shrimp cocktail with red sauce, a small salad, or a cup of soup. As usual, try to avoid cream-based soups and go easy on high-fat salad dressings.

What about salad or soup and half a sandwich? Would your child enjoy a cup of minestrone and half a turkey sandwich; or a green salad and half a lean roast beef sandwich? Other reasonable sandwich choices might be grilled chicken or ham, but not if they're slathered with mayonnaise or topped with cheese, bacon, or avocado. Another concern about sandwiches is what comes on the plate with them: chips, French fries, and potato salad are all high in calories. Sometimes coleslaw is better, if it's not too creamy. Or ask for a fruit cup instead.

Although American-style restaurant menus vary widely, chances are you'll find a hamburger or two on every one. The key to ordering hamburgers is to watch the size and the toppings. Smaller is better than larger; and low-fat toppings, such as lettuce, tomato, onions, mustard, ketchup, and barbecue sauce, are preferable to mayonnaise, cheese, bacon, or avocado.

When it comes to entrees, the following terms will tip you off that the dish is high-fat and high-calorie: buttery, butter sauce, fried, crispy, creamed, cream sauce, gravy, hollandaise, au gratin, cheese sauce, or marinated in oil.

More appropriate entrees include stir-fry dishes or broiled or grilled fish or chicken. Vegetables are good accompaniments, as are starches, such as baked potatoes or rice. Ask the waiter if you're not sure how a menu item is cooked.

Italian-Style Restaurant

What child doesn't like pizza? And if you order carefully, pizza can be the foundation of a nutritious, moderate-fat meal away from home. The two main considerations with pizza are the same as for hamburgers: size and toppings. Although pizzas are generally shared, don't automatically order an extra-large. Nobody needs those extra slices staring at them, just begging to be eaten.

When it comes to toppings, less is more. Most children are happy with plain cheese pizza. But if you would like some extras, choose among such low-fat options as mushrooms, green peppers, sliced tomatoes, garlic, onions, chicken, and pineapple. Steer clear of high-fat additions, such as extra cheese, olives, pepperoni, sausage, bacon, meatballs, and prosciutto. And definitely don't get the house pizza with "everything" on it.

A mixed green salad with low-fat dressing or a modest amount of vinaigrette is a good accompaniment to a pizza. However, a Caesar salad, with its fried croutons and cheesy dressing, or a spinach salad with bacon and egg contains too much fat for a few leaves of lettuce.

But there's more to Italian restaurants than just pizza. Italian soups are often filling and low fat. A bowl of minestrone, tortellini in broth, or pasta e fagioli (pasta and bean soup) might be a satisfying entree for your child—especially if accompanied by a green salad and a piece of crusty bread.

All pastas are low in fat, until the chef ladles on the sauce. The key to sauces is mostly in the color: red sauces (tomato/basil, marinara, Bolognese) are generally lowest in fat; followed by green (pesto or Florentine), which tend to be higher-fat; and white sauces (Alfredo, carbonara, or cheese), which are the highest in fat. The exception to the color rule may be white clam sauce, which is sometimes a low-fat, white-wine- or broth-based sauce.

But even with low-fat toppings, pasta can be a high-calorie entree because the portion sizes are often so large. Perhaps your child would be satisfied with an appetizer portion, especially if the sauce contains some protein, such as meatballs, chicken, or seafood.

Cheese can add a lot of fat and calories to Italian food. A little sprinkling of Parmesan on a plate of spaghetti is okay, but it doesn't need to blanket the pasta like a heavy snow. Also, be aware that baked pasta dishes, such as cannelloni, manicotti, and lasagna, usually ooze with high-fat cheese. Gnocchi are a little higher in fat than noodles, but if you order them with a low-fat sauce, they are good for variety.

With meat dishes, the sauce tells the story again: chicken cacciatore, primavera, or marinara are probably good choices. More likely to be higher in fat are piccata, marsala, Parmigiana, or pesto.

For dessert, Italian ices are a no-fat sweet to end the meal. However, most traditional Italian desserts, such as spumoni, cannoli, gelato, and tiramisu, are high fat and very high calorie and are better reserved for special treats.

Chinese-Style Restaurants

The good news is that many Chinese dishes emphasize vegetables and starches—rice and noodles. The bad news is that some cooking techniques can turn these low-fat ingredients into high-fat dishes. So instead of such appetizers as fried won ton, egg rolls, pot stickers, spring rolls, spare ribs, or fried shrimp, order a bowl of soup for the table: hot and sour, sizzling rice, or won ton are good choices. Another possibility is to get an order of mu-shu chicken or vegetables —enough for each person to have one rolled pancake as an appetizer.

You'll find many low-fat, nutritious choices for main dishes. Look for entrees that contain vegetables, chicken, seafood, or steamed tofu—all low-fat. Look *out* for dishes containing duck, pork, or nuts, such as cashews or peanuts, which are all high-fat.

Cooking techniques can make all the difference in whether low-fat ingredients remain low-fat by the time they make it to your table.

Choose dishes that are simmered, steamed, or roasted for the lowest amount of fat at a Chinese restaurant. Stir-frying is a bit higher in fat, so you might ask that the chef go easy on the oil. You'll be tipped off to high-fat preparations by words such as deep fried, breaded, and crispy. Although sweet and sour dishes don't say "fried," the pork or chicken is nearly always breaded and deep fried before it's put in the sauce. If you're unsure about the preparation, ask the waiter.

When it comes to the rice, try to choose steamed instead of fried. And lo-mein or chow-mein noodle dishes are lower in fat than pan-fried noodles, which are, in turn, lower in fat than crispy noodles.

Most people order several dishes for the table and eat family style. Perhaps the most difficult thing at a Chinese restaurant is to refrain from ordering too many different items. Don't let your eyes or hunger cause you to over-order. You can always ask for another dish later on in the meal. The next hardest thing is to get family members to stop eating when they're satisfied and not clean off all the serving plates. One strategy is to be prompt about asking for cartons to pack up the take-homes. Don't wait until there's nothing left to take home.

Fruit and fortune cookies are light, refreshing desserts. Skip the almond cookies and custards.

Mexican-Style Restaurants

Mexican restaurants are among the most challenging places to order a low-fat meal. If your family loves Mexican food, you'll have to do the best you can, because the truth is, most dishes on the menu are high fat and high calorie.

It starts from the minute you sit down to the table and find a bowl of deep fried tortilla chips and salsa. Keep the salsa, but ask your waiter if you can have a basket of warm, soft tortillas instead of the chips. You may have to pay more, but you'll be saving loads of extra fat calories.

And you can save both money and calories by skipping appetizers such as quesadillas, nachos, chili con queso, or guacamole and chips. However, the appetizer section might be a good place if your child likes soup, such as black bean or gazpacho. You also might find chili con carne, which could serve as a child-sized entree.

But, most likely, you will want to simply order a main course.

Steer clear of the combination plates, unless you're planning to share. They are just too big. The next consideration is what type of dish to order. The lower-fat items at a Mexican restaurant are likely to be soft tacos, enchiladas, burritos, tamales, and fajitas—made with chicken. But in order to keep them low fat, refrain from smothering them in guacamole or sour cream. When the tortillas are fried, the fat content shoots way up, so it's best to avoid chimichangas, flautas, and crisp tacos.

Beans and rice are common side dishes with a Mexican meal. The rice is fine, but if whole beans are available, they're a much-lower-fat accompaniment than refried beans. If you can order à la carte for your child, a good, low-fat dinner would be a soft chicken taco or chicken fajitas with rice and salad.

Breakfast Time

Some families eat breakfast or brunch in a restaurant as a relaxing weekend tradition. Others find themselves grabbing breakfast at a fast-food restaurant during the week as a matter of survival.

Low-fat breakfast selections at fast-food places are limited. The best choices are toast, English muffins, or bagels with jelly; orange juice; and fat-free or low-fat milk. When it comes to the various "breakfast sandwiches" offered at most fast-food establishments, you have to be careful. About the lowest fat you can get is an egg on an English muffin, with or without a slice of Canadian bacon. But breakfast sandwiches that include sausage, bacon, or cheese or are served on a biscuit or croissant are automatically high in fat and calories.

Breakfast or brunch in a restaurant generally provides greater opportunities for low-fat choices. Fruit and fruit juice are always on the menu and can take the edge off a child's hunger while waiting for the rest of the meal. Also, hot and cold cereals usually are available.

Pancakes and waffles need not be high in fat—that is, if they're topped with fruit or a little syrup (not butter *and* syrup, or whipped cream *and* fruit) and if they don't share the plate with bacon, sausage, or ham. Canadian bacon is a moderate-fat breakfast meat. But don't be fooled by muffins. They are often as high in fat and calories as doughnuts, Danish pastries, or scones.

If the choice is eggs, perhaps one egg, instead of two, scrambled or poached would be acceptable to your child, with the addition of toast, fruit, and milk. This breakfast is much lower in fat and calories than fried eggs with bacon and hash brown potatoes.

Fast-Food Restaurants

Fast-food restaurants are kid-pleasers and parent-savers. They're places to get predictable, reasonably priced food that your child will like. And despite their abundance of high-fat items, many now offer a variety of lower-fat lunch and dinner choices for children.

The special children's meal at fast-food restaurants usually includes a choice of hamburger, cheeseburger, or chicken nuggets; a small order of French fries; and a choice of soda, milk, or juice. The lowest-fat meal providing the best nutrition would be the hamburger, low-fat milk, and fries. In case you were wondering why we didn't pick the chicken, that's because it's deep-fat fried, making it higher in fat and calories than the hamburger.

If your child doesn't insist on the special meal, he could have a small salad instead of fries. But watch out for the salad dressing. If he likes the low-fat offering, great. If not, try a vinaigrette type and help him use just enough—not the whole packet.

Another approach at fast-food restaurants is to allow one treat per visit. She can have either a soda or fries or cheese on her burger. Not all three. Sharing is another strategy. Perhaps two children can share a small order of fries or onion rings. Milkshakes might also be appropriate for splitting—although fast-food shakes are generally low in fat, they range in calories from 300 to 400.

A lot of the calories in a fast-food meal can come from soda. As the size increases, so do the empty calories. For example, at our local fast-food restaurant, a small soda has 150 calories. With a large, at 310, you more than double the calories, and a supersize drink has a whopping 410 calories.

Some fast-food restaurants are responding to their customers' requests for low-fat options by providing lower-fat hamburgers and plain baked potatoes. Just keep in mind that while a baked potato has no fat, if you load it up with sour cream, butter, and/or cheese, you turn it into a high-fat dish. Would your child go for a baked potato topped with salsa, chili, or cottage cheese?

Other good low-fat, fast-food choices are sandwiches, salads, or fajitas made with broiled, grilled, or roasted chicken. But be suspicious of any chicken dish that doesn't specify how it's cooked. Chances are it's deep-fat fried. Even innocent-sounding chicken tenders, chicken fillets, or chicken strips are probably breaded and fried. If you're not sure, ask. The same is true for fish. We're not aware of any fast-food fish sandwich that isn't fried. For this reason, a fast-food roast beef sandwich is generally lower in fat and calories than the fish sandwich.

If you frequent a particular establishment, ask for their nutritional information brochure. That's the best way to make informed choices. And if your regular fast-food place has a salad bar, refer to the section later in this chapter for tips on surfing the salad bar.

Convenience Stores

When you need food fast, you don't always have to go to a fast-food restaurant. Many convenience stores offer a variety of quick picks. The trick is to get past the high-fat, sugary temptations at the counter. But if you poke around, you'll find some acceptable quick lunch or snack possibilities for your child.

For the same money as a bag of chips and a soda, you can buy a yogurt and some fruit. Here are some suggestions for single-serving, eat-in-the-car foods for those days when you and your child are on the go:

- String cheese
- Yogurt
- Fruit—fresh or fruit cup
- Raisins
- Pretzels
- Bagels
- Low-fat energy or granola bar (read the label to be sure it's low calorie)
- Wrapped sandwiches (look for turkey, chicken, or lean roast beef)
- Fruit juice
- Low-fat milk

Vending Machines

A vending machine is not the likeliest place to find a low-fat snack, but some do have items that fall into the healthy category. You'll still find plenty of candy and sodas, but you might be surprised to find that yogurt, fresh fruit, pretzels, low-fat granola bars, soups, low-fat milk, and juice can come out of a machine, too. Prepared sandwiches are sometimes offered in vending machines. If given the option, try to steer your child to a turkey, chicken, or roast beef sandwich, which will generally be lower in fat than tuna or egg salad.

Salad Bars

Salad bars are everywhere, not only in traditional restaurants, but also in fast-food places and grocery stores. And that's good news when you're on the go and looking for a nutritious, low-fat lunch or dinner for you and your child. If you're making the salad to accompany a meal, stick to a small bowl and include just vegetables.

If you're using the salad bar to create a meal in a bowl, don't forget to include adequate protein. Low-fat choices include chicken, turkey, tuna (not tuna salad), cottage cheese, tofu, and beans, such as garbanzo or kidney.

Most vegetables offered at the salad bar can be scooped generously into your child's bowl: lettuce, sprouts, beets, carrots, mushrooms, tomatoes, and broccoli are some of the choices. Starchy vegetables, such as corn and peas, are good, too; as is fruit, such as pineapple, pears, and peaches. Don't pile on the prepared salads, such as potato, pasta, or macaroni salad or coleslaw. They are loaded with mayonnaise. But perhaps a small spoonful of his one favorite would be appropriate.

The toppings at the end of the line can derail your best intentions for a low-fat salad. Bacon bits, cheese, sunflower seeds, olives, chopped egg, and croutons are all almost pure fat. Salad dressing, as always, is a bit tricky. However, most salad bars do offer reduced-fat dressings. Another option would be to help your child use the vinegar and oil cruets—to apply a generous amount of vinegar and a modest amount of oil. Or use a small amount of his favorite dressing.

A piece of bread helps round out a salad bar meal, especially if your child didn't choose many starchy vegetables to put on his salad.

School or Day Care

The best strategy to help your child eat low-calorie foods at day care is to pack appropriate snacks and meals for her to take with her. If this isn't possible, because of your schedule or day care regulations, talk to the day care provider and see if you can influence him or her to serve healthy, low-fat snacks and meals for all the children. You might want to talk to some of the other parents to see if they will lend their support.

Your school-age child is probably more concerned about how his lunch bag or lunch box looks on the outside, but we know that it's what's inside that counts. The sandwich is the most popular item for a portable lunch. Whether it's on a roll, between two slices of bread, or in a pita pocket, sandwiches are easy to make and easy to eat.

Three things distinguish a healthy, low-fat sandwich from its high-fat cousin: the choice of filling, spread, and accessories. We've provided some suggestions for low-fat choices in each category to help get you started. It's up to you to be creative in your combinations and to think up other low-fat sandwich ingredients.

Fillings	Spreads	Accessories
Water-pack tuna salad	Reduced-fat mayonnaise	Sprouts
Chicken	Fat-free mayonnaise	Sliced cucumbers
Turkey	Cranberry sauce	Lettuce
Reduced-fat or fat-free cheese	Reduced-fat margarine	Tomatoes
Lean ham	Mustard	Pickles
Reduced-fat peanut butter	Jelly	Bananas
Lean roast beef	Barbecue sauce	Sliced green pepper

If your child doesn't like sandwiches, pick a low-fat protein source and match it with an appropriate fruit or vegetable and a starch. For example, a carton of yogurt goes well with a banana and some pretzels. Cottage cheese can be paired with fruit and low-fat crackers. A couple of ounces of reduced-fat cheese can be accompanied by an apple and a small French roll. Favorite low-fat leftovers from dinner can also be popular at lunch.

Entertainment Activities

The food concessions at ball games, movies, and amusement parks try to convince us that we can't be having fun unless we're eating their high-fat, high-calorie foods.

If your family is drawn to the popcorn and candy counter on the way into the theater, try agreeing on some limits before you go to the movies. Instead of an individual box of popcorn for each family member, plan to buy a slightly larger box for the whole family to share. If your child really wants candy, tell her she has to decide between candy and popcorn. She can't have both. If she chooses the candy, give her the opportunity to pick something small at a store on the way to the theater. Pure sugar candies, such as gummy bears or jelly beans, are low-fat choices but are still high in calories. Refer to our chart on page 119 for more ideas. But remember, a *small* chocolate bar is still better than the jumbo candy bars and oversized boxes of candy they sell at the movies.

The sodas in movies keep getting larger and larger. If your child insists on soda, make it a small cup—even that will add 150 to 200 empty calories.

If visits to ball games and amusement parks are special occasions, you can let your child enjoy his favorite treats without much concern. However, if your family has season tickets to the baseball park, you'll be better off packing a low-fat lunch and telling your child he can pick one treat at the game—a small soda or maybe a small bag of caramel corn or an ice cream.

Eating away from home is a fact of life. Avoiding restaurants is not an appropriate way to help your overweight child. Instead, use eating out as an opportunity to help her learn how to manage her eating wherever life takes her.

PART IV

Focus on Fitness

18

Off the Couch!

WHOEVER COINED THE PHRASE "couch potato" managed, in two little words, to portray both the state of being inactive and the effects of a sedentary lifestyle. *Couch* because we tend to be conspicuously inactive on the living room sofa—lounging, napping, or watching television. And what kind of inert vegetable are we most likely to resemble if we spend too much time lying around on the couch—not a string bean or a carrot but a *potato*. Get the picture? That's why we want to help you get the potatoes in your house *off* the couch and engaged in more active pursuits.

Is Progress Making Our Children Chubbier?

Why are more American children overweight today than at any other time in our history? We think the most important reason is that children are less active now than ever before.

In the past one hundred years, amazing technological achievements have changed our way of life. These advances have streamlined the way we do work, made it easier to go from place to place, and created an abundance of entertainment options that require no active participation. The widespread use of two modern inventions— the television and the automobile—have contributed significantly to the decrease in physical activity among adults and children.

The Trouble With Television

Children in the United States spend more time watching television than they do involved in any other activity except sleep. The average

American child watches twenty-two to twenty-eight hours of television a week. Take a look at the Activity Assessment you filled out on page 36 to see how much time your child spends watching TV. If her average is anywhere near the *national* average, there's a lot of room for improvement.

Watching television is like eating high-fat food. In moderate amounts, it doesn't cause obesity, but when consumed in excessive quantities, it can contribute significantly to a child's being overweight. One study of adolescents found that, for each hour of television viewing, there was a 2 percent increase in the prevalence of obesity.

Television viewing promotes weight gain in several ways. First, it is one of the most sedentary activities a child can engage in. Surprisingly, a research study comparing the difference between the energy expended by girls watching television and the same girls lying down resting (but not sleeping) found that, when the girls were watching television, they burned significantly fewer calories than when they were resting.

If watching television were simply a sedentary activity, we might think of it as equivalent to a child getting a few extra hours of sleep a day. But there's an added dimension to television viewing that makes it more hazardous to an overweight child than dozing off on the couch. We're talking about the relentless commercials that bombard your child with enticing images of high-fat, high-sugar foods. These advertisements for sugary cereals, candy, and fast foods are extremely effective, prompting your child to beg you to buy the items for him or, if he's old enough, to purchase them for himself.

Food commercials have an additional effect. They make us want to eat. Even if we don't have immediate access to the particular food being advertised, the images make us crave something equally tasty. And to make these cravings even harder to resist, the commercial breaks provide us with enough time to run to the kitchen for a high-calorie munchie without missing a minute of our favorite program.

Watching television is a reasonable way for children to relax. However, spending too much time in front of the TV limits the amount of time available for more active pursuits. The President's Council on Physical Fitness recommends that children engage in one hour of vigorous activity per day. A good way to make time for exercise in a sedentary child's schedule is to reduce his television viewing time.

As with all changes to a child's routine, reducing TV time should be done gradually. First, consider how much time your child spends watching television. If it's more than two hours a day, try reducing the amount by thirty minutes. At the same time, try to substitute a more physical activity that your child enjoys. See chapter 20 for ways to make exercise fun. After your child has adjusted to watching less television, try cutting TV viewing by another thirty minutes a day. Continue with this process over time, until you have achieved a level that is acceptable to both you and your child, one that allows ample time for schoolwork and physical activity.

Get Out of the Car

Cars are a convenience to most, a necessity to some, and a habit to many of us. How often do you and your child hop in the car to go someplace you could have easily walked to? Chances are you don't even stop to consider using foot power instead of horsepower. That is, unless you live in a city so congested that it's impractical to use a car for short trips.

In any case, we're not recommending that you trade in the family car for bicycles or walking shoes. What we are suggesting is that you consider ways for your child and your family to get where you need to go while burning a few extra calories along the way.

If you give it some thought, you probably can come up with a number of opportunities to leave the car in the garage. If you currently give your child a ride to school, could she walk instead? If she's too rushed in the morning to walk, how about giving her a ride to school and letting her walk home? If safety is an issue, maybe she could walk with a sibling or friend. If it's too far to walk to school, is she old enough and is it safe enough for her to ride her bike?

Another idea is to invite your child to walk or ride his bike to the store with you if you're not buying a lot of heavy items. If the trip is less than half a mile each way, you can walk there and back in scarcely more time than it would take to drive and park the car. And on a bicycle, even a two-mile round trip is time efficient.

If your home is miles away from school and stores, you still have some options for getting out of the car. Perhaps when you drive to the mall, you could park as far away from your destination as possible, instead of circling around looking for the closest spot. If your child gives you a quizzical look, explain that it's good exercise.

Can you think of any other ways to help your child get some extra exercise while going from here to there?

What Happened to Physical Education?

Before widespread cuts to education budgets, the effects of television watching and automobile riding could at least be offset somewhat by physical activity during the school day. Children used to get a reasonable amount of exercise playing in the school yard at recess and taking daily physical education classes. Physical education is now considered by many schools in our country as a luxury to be diminished or completely eliminated from school curricula.

You could try to lobby your school or school district to reinstate or expand its physical education program. But perhaps a more immediate solution is to counteract the sedentary hours your child spends at school with after-school programs and weekend activities that involve exercise. We will discuss this in more detail in the next chapter.

Fourteen Fabulous Facts About Exercise

Regardless of why your child spends too little time being active— whether it's too much television, too much reliance on Mom or Dad to drive her everywhere, or too little physical education at school— now is the time to help her overcome her inertia and get moving.

We know that changing sedentary habits may take a lot of effort on your part as well as your child's. You may even be thinking, "If I help my child by preparing nutritious, low-fat food, do I really need to help him be more physically active, too?" The answer is "yes" and we can give you fourteen good reasons why.

1. *Exercise combined with a healthy diet is the most effective method of weight control.* There's only one way to lose a pound of fat—consume 3,500 fewer calories than your body requires to carry

out the activities of daily living. You can do this by eating fewer calories or by burning more calories. But time and again, research demonstrates that a combination of diet modifications and increased physical activity offers the most effective approach to weight loss and the best hope for long-term weight control.

2. *Exercise burns extra calories while you're doing it.* Although exercising doesn't burn a huge amount of calories, it's better than sitting still or, as we've seen, watching television. Watching television burns perhaps one calorie per minute, whereas light physical activities, such as Ping-Pong or volleyball, can burn four calories per minute. Moderate exercise, such as brisk walking or biking, may burn seven calories per minute; while heavy exercise, such as jogging or skipping rope, could burn ten or more calories each minute.

3. *Exercise helps your body burn extra calories even after you finish.* Exercise temporarily increases one's basal metabolic rate (BMR), the rate at which your body burns calories while at rest. The higher your BMR, the more calories you need just to exist. During exercise, your BMR increases and can remain elevated for a period of time, depending upon the intensity and duration of the exercise session. For example, one's BMR can stay elevated for six to twenty-four hours after thirty minutes of moderate exercise. So even though some calories are burned during exercise, of greater benefit is the increase in BMR that helps burn extra calories for hours after one is physically active.

4. *Exercise maintains lean body mass, which also increases metabolism (BMR).* By helping to maintain lean body mass (muscle), regular exercise can increase BMR on a more long-term basis. The more muscle you have, the more calories you burn just sitting around. This is important because a weight loss plan that includes only changes in diet will cause a loss in *muscle* as well as fat. This reduction in muscle, in turn, slows down your body's metabolism, making it harder to keep the weight off. However, when exercise is part of the program, most of one's calorie-burning muscle tissue is retained.

5. *Exercise helps decrease body fat.* Exercising helps build muscle, which is the part of your body that burns calories. In fact, every pound of muscle requires fifty calories per day to stay alive, whereas fat uses no calories. When your muscles don't get enough calories from the food you eat, they will burn some of your stored fat for

energy. Therefore, the more muscle you build with exercise, the more fat you're able to burn.

6. *Exercise improves physical fitness.* A child who is sedentary may get out of breath walking up a hill or become overly tired from moderate physical activity. An exercise program that starts slowly and gradually builds up in duration and intensity can improve physical fitness and allow a child to feel good about how his body functions.

7. *Exercise can help control appetite.* Although this is not a universal phenomenon, most people report that exercise makes them feel less hungry. Contrary to popular opinion, exercise does not cause people to eat more.

8. *Exercise can take a child's mind off eating.* Most forms of exercise are not performed in the kitchen or in other locations where food is easily accessible. Therefore, exercising can be an effective way to keep food out of sight and, therefore, out of mind.

9. *Changing a child's exercise patterns may be easier than changing her food habits.* If a child is having trouble changing the food behaviors that are contributing to her weight problem, it may be more effective to help her increase her level of physical activity instead. Not only can exercise help burn up some extra calories, it also can give a child a feeling of being successful at something. The success of becoming more physically fit or achieving incremental exercise goals may give her enough confidence to start working on the food-related issues.

10. *Exercise can reduce stress.* This is particularly helpful if a child has the tendency to eat when feeling stressed. Exercise can take his mind off his troubles. It also helps work tension out of the body and provides a physical release from stress.

11. *Exercise can increase self-esteem.* Physical activity can give a child a real sense of well-being. Becoming more physically fit helps a child feel more confident about her ability to move her body. And the gradual improvement in coordination skills that comes with practice can also give a child a sense of accomplishment that will enhance her self-esteem.

12. *Exercise can increase a child's social contact and improve social skills.* A child who joins a team, takes a class, or simply participates in neighborhood activities has a greater opportunity to meet other children. This increased interaction can help a child reduce

loneliness, learn how to get along better with his peers, as well as have fun.

13. *Exercise combats boredom.* A child won't be bored if she's busy. So if your child tends to eat when she's bored, being more physically active can help reduce her tendency to eat when she's not really hungry.

14. *Exercise can become a lifelong, healthy habit.* If your child has happy experiences with exercise as a youngster, he will carry that positive feeling with him for the rest of his life. But if your efforts to encourage your child to exercise are too intense or otherwise inappropriate, they can backfire, causing your child to develop negative feelings about exercise. A research study found that sedentary adults are more likely to have had unfavorable experiences related to exercise as adolescents than the adults who engage in regular exercise. That's why we're devoting a whole chapter to the subject of making exercise fun for your child. If children view physical activity as a positive experience, they are more likely to keep exercising throughout their lives.

Dispelling Exercise Myths

With all of the benefits of physical activity, why don't more children, and adults, exercise regularly? Perhaps you and your child have fallen prey to one of the many misconceptions about exercise. Let's dispel some of these myths, so they are no longer barriers to getting off the couch.

Myth 1: Exercising makes you eat more.

Fact: While not everyone experiences a decrease in appetite during or after exercise, moderate physical activity has *not* been shown to increase appetite among people who are trying to reduce or control weight. However, some people think that a bout of exercise burns off so many calories that they can overindulge—this is Myth 6.

Myth 2: No pain, no gain.

Fact: Especially when it comes to children, the phrase should be: "If there's pain, there will be no gain." Exercise has to be moderate and fun: The intensity and duration should be increased only gradually and at a pace that is comfortable and enjoyable for your child. Overdoing it can cause sore muscles, which may discourage your youngster from exercising again.

Myth 3: It's useless to exercise if you can't exercise thirty minutes at a time.

Fact: Any activity, however mild or short in duration, is valuable. Especially for an out-of-shape or overweight child, begin adding exercise slowly. Even ten minutes of walking a day may be appropriate at first, with five minutes per session added each week to gradually build endurance.

Myth 4: Some people were just not meant to be athletic.

Fact: While some people aren't as well-coordinated as others, or have no desire to become competitive athletes, every individual, child or adult, can be "active and fit," which just happens to be the definition of "athletic."

Myth 5: Jogging a mile burns more calories than walking a mile.

Fact: You burn the same number of calories jogging or walking a mile. It merely takes less time to jog the distance. If your child is just beginning to be more active, walking is a much gentler, but still effective, way to start. Over time, she can work up to jogging or running if she wants.

Unfortunately, we also need to dispel two exercise myths everyone wishes were true.

Myth 6: If you exercise, you can eat all you want.

Fact: This may be true for some marathon runners or other elite athletes; but for us mere mortals, exercise simply allows us to eat a bit more without gaining weight. If the goal is weight loss, consuming fewer calories while burning more through exercise is still the most effective approach.

Myth 7: You can reduce specific parts of your body by doing many repetitions of exercises designed for those regions.

Fact: Spot reducing is not possible. Leg lifts don't melt fat from our thighs and sit-ups can't make a bulging tummy flat. Depending mostly on genetics, fat will be reduced from where it was put on last, from the area with the most fat, or uniformly from all parts of the body. Exercising a group of muscles at a specific spot on the body can tone and firm them. But it can't make your body get rid of the excess fat that sits on top of these muscles.

Inactivity and Obesity: the Chicken and the Egg

Some experts assert that lack of exercise is the major cause of childhood obesity. Others maintain that children who are overweight exercise less because they tire easily or are embarrassed about their bodies. Regardless of which came first, the sedentary habits or the overweight child, there's one solution—to get moving. How you approach this aspect of your child's effort to manage his weight is vitally important. In the upcoming chapters we'll help you target ways to help your child *enjoy* getting off the couch.

19

Every Little Activity Helps

DENNIS THE MENACE IS THE EPITOME of an active child, climbing trees, pulling his little red wagon through the neighborhood, playing with his dog Ruff, and escaping from Mr. Wilson. He's always on the go, yet nothing he does would be considered "exercise."

Exercise is defined as "activity for the purpose of training or developing the body" or "bodily exertion for the sake of health." We doubt that Dennis is thinking about his health as he dashes about—his only objective is having fun.

While regular exercise should be the long-range goal for your child, if she's currently a couch potato, the first step is simply encouraging her to replace some of her inactivity with activity.

Exercise is a specialized kind of activity. Your child might enjoy PE classes or team sports, but for many sedentary children, organized exercise programs are not necessarily the best place to start. The intensity of some forms of exercise may make a child who is out of shape feel uncomfortable. Similarly, the competitive nature of team sports may be threatening for a youngster who doesn't feel athletic.

In contrast to exercise, activity is defined simply as "the quality or state of being active." Therefore, anything that gets your child moving is an activity. Activities tend to be more flexible and less structured than exercise—and often more fun.

It Doesn't Have to Be Exercise

For the purposes of weight control, activities that burn calories and help speed up metabolism are the most desirable. But anything that can pry a child away from the television set or computer screen is a step in the right direction. Here are some pastimes that you might not immediately think of as physical activities:

- Building a fort
- Flying a kite
- Making a snowman
- Planting a garden
- Playing with the dog
- Raking leaves
- Running through the sprinklers
- Shoveling snow
- Washing the car

We're not trying to fool you into thinking that raking leaves once a week or playing with the dog after school is enough activity to help your child significantly with her weight. However, light activities such as these are still useful. First, any physical activity is better than sitting around watching television. Second, mild activities are a gentle way to ease your child into more challenging activities or regular exercise. And third, even for a child who plays sports or participates in other kinds of exercise, moderate activities can add variety and burn a few extra calories.

Add More Activity Gradually

As with changes in food habits, changes in activity patterns must be made slowly. If an activity is fun and moderate enough not to cause your child discomfort, he's more likely to want to do it again. However, if the activity is too extreme or unpleasant, he is apt to revert back to his sedentary ways.

We mentioned in the last chapter that the President's Council on Physical Fitness recommends that children engage in one hour of vigorous activity per day. We want to point out that it says "vigorous activity," not "exercise." The council must have understood that activities don't have to conform to the definition of exercise in order to be beneficial for a child's health.

If one hour a day seems unrealistic, consider half an hour of activity as an intermediate goal to work toward. When thirty minutes becomes a natural part of her life, she can start adding activities to get closer to one hour. See the example below that shows how an hour of activity might fit into a child's day. You'll notice that Active Alice's schedule includes activities and exercise that add up to one hour of *moving* around, while Sedentary Sally spends the same hour *sitting* around.

Active Alice	Sedentary Sally
Walks to and from school (20 minutes)	Gets a ride to and from school
Plays tag at recess (10 minutes)	Sits on bench and talks to her friend during recess
Rides bike after school with her friend (20 minutes) Walks the dog (10 minutes)	Watches television after school until it's time for dinner

How Often, How Long, How Hard?

There are three variables that can be used to describe any physical activity or exercise:

Frequency: how often one engages in the activity. Frequency ranges from never, to a few times a week, to every day, to several times a day.

Duration: how long the exercise or activity lasts. This can be from one minute, to an hour, to several hours at a time.

Intensity: how hard the person exerts him or herself throughout the exercise or activity session. Walking on a level block is less intense than walking uphill.

In general, the greater the frequency, duration, and intensity of exercise, the more likely a person is to derive the many benefits we discussed in the last chapter. For example, John, who walks for an hour a day at a pace of four miles an hour, is getting more weight-control benefits than Victor, who walks for half an hour, twice a week, at a pace of three miles an hour. John's weekly exercise program involves greater frequency (seven times a week, compared to two times), greater intensity (four mph instead of three mph), and greater duration (sixty minutes instead of thirty minutes at a time). This isn't to say that Victor's activity is worthless. After all, he's doing much better than Sedentary Sally. Remember, every little activity helps, but the more the better.

There are many different approaches to getting more exercise, but we think it's easiest and most effective for a sedentary child to get used to frequency first. And it's not unreasonable for a child to do some kind of physical activity every day.

When we were growing up, our parents encouraged us to go out and play after school. The reality is that it's not always safe for children to play outside alone. However, that's no excuse for a child not to be able to engage in some kind of physical activity every day, whether it's inside dancing to a music tape or video, or outside playing basketball with his brother or taking a walk with Mom.

The reason we suggest starting with frequency is that if your child gets used to doing something active every day, it will become a healthy habit, just like brushing her teeth. Once it's a habit, the duration and intensity can be gradually increased. And, as we saw with Active Alice, eventually your child will have days when she's doing a variety of activities and exercises. On other days it might be one long activity, such as a hike or an afternoon spent walking around the zoo.

Just one reminder: Although the goal is for your child to get some exercise every day, it may take a while to get into the habit. Even when it's part of the routine, there will be days when your child doesn't do anything. And just as there are no bad foods, a day without exercise isn't a bad day—it's just a day without exercise.

Increase the Benefits of Physical Activity

If being active is new to your child, be sure she starts with activities that are modest in duration and intensity. For example, your child's first activity might be to walk the dog to the park and back (fifteen minutes) once a day. When that has become a comfortable routine, the duration could be increased by walking the dog to another destination, farther away, so that it takes thirty minutes to walk round trip. Another option would be to increase the intensity of the exercise. Your child could walk for fifteen minutes on a different route that includes a little hill. A third option is to do the original walk to the park and back, but increase the frequency to twice a day.

While moderation is essential at the beginning, if the frequency, duration, or intensity of the activities stays too low, your child won't be getting the weight-control benefits that more regular, vigorous exercise would provide. Over time, she will need to increase frequency, duration, and intensity in order to have a significant impact on her weight.

To illustrate how this might work, we're going to tell you about three children who are somewhat active, but who all could be getting more benefit from their activities.

Frank is a weekend athlete. He plays basketball on Saturday mornings and goes bike riding with his father almost every Sunday. But during the week, it's school, homework, and television. Frank's weekend activities are great. They are intense enough to burn some calories and they last long enough for some metabolic improvement. But these weekend benefits can't carry him through the week. We suggest adding frequency to Frank's exercise program, until he's doing something every day. Perhaps he could ride his bike to and from school, or maybe he could join a team that has practice or games after school.

Irene participates in organized activities every day. She has soccer practice after school and games on Saturday. She often plays softball with her friends on Sunday. But a closer look finds that she's the goalie on the soccer team, so she spends most of her time standing around waiting for her ten seconds of action. She plays left field on the softball team, so she does a lot of standing around there, too. The only time she's really moving is when she hits the ball and gets to run around the bases. To get more benefit from her activities, Irene needs to increase the intensity of her exercise sessions. The frequency (every day) and duration (one to two hours) are fine. If she likes soccer, maybe she can ask to be moved to a position where she gets to run more during the game. And if she doesn't want to give up softball, perhaps she can ride her bike to and from the games. If she would consider a different weekend activity, hiking or roller-blading might be good alternatives that require a bit more effort than softball.

Ricky walks to school every day and spends weekend afternoons in-line skating with his best friend. The school Ricky went to last year was two miles away, so it took him forty minutes to walk each way. However, his new school is just three blocks from his house, so his trip only takes five minutes each way. Ricky's activities are of good intensity and he does do something every day. However, by decreasing the duration of his walk to school by more than an hour a day, he's lost out on five hours of exercise a week. If Ricky likes to walk, perhaps he could go for a walk after school for an hour before he starts his homework. Or maybe he'd prefer to take a class or join a team.

How Active Is Your Child?

Looking back at your child's Activity Assessment on page 36 and using the descriptions below, consider how you would define your child's level of activity over the past three to six months.

Inactive: He watches television, reads, surfs the Internet or does homework after school. He rides to and from school in a car or bus and doesn't play any extracurricular sports.

Occasionally active: She prefers sedentary activities, such as watching TV, reading, e-mailing friends or playing video games, but sometimes plays outside.

Moderately active: He becomes involved in physical activities when they are available and if he enjoys them.

Active: She takes the initiative to participate in physical activities. She does some form of activity every day, and three days a week she is involved in vigorous exercise.

Very active: He participates regularly in school and extracurricular sports. He has a lot of energy and dislikes sedentary activities.

If your child is less than "Active," take a closer look at her Assessment and see if you can identify ways to improve the frequency, intensity, or duration of your child's physical activities.

Question 1 on the Activity Assessment asked you to keep track of how much time your child and other family members spend watching television. We've mentioned the merits of trying to cut back on television viewing, including making time in your child's schedule for more physical activities. However, you'll need to take into consideration how your child's viewing time compares to that of other family members. If he's watching more than anyone else, you could try limiting his time so it's more in line with the rest of the family. But if everyone's watching too much television, maybe the whole family should cut down.

In addition to television, consider how much time your child spends playing games that are sedentary, whether they're video games, computer games, or board games. These passive activities can add up and infringe on exercise time as well.

Questions 2 and 3 asked about whether your child walks or bikes to school. If she's not getting to school under her own steam, and it's reasonable and safe for her to do so, now is a good time to start. If she's already getting back and forth to school on her own, maybe the distance isn't great enough to provide enough benefit. In that case, try to help her discover other activities to add to her day.

Question 4 was about your child's participation in physical education at school. We know that PE might not be available, but if it is, maybe he could take one of the classes. Ask what activities are available and help him pick one that he would enjoy. But be aware, PE classes can be deceptive when it comes to intensity and duration. One study found that the average forty-minute PE class provided youngsters with only three minutes of vigorous activity.

Question 5 concerned organized after-school or weekend activities. Consider frequency (how many times a week) and duration (for how long). If your child isn't involved in after-school activities, you might start by finding out if her school has any programs. If none are offered, check out community agencies close to where you live. If there are no organized programs in your area, perhaps there is a bike path where you could take your child after school, or where she could ride with a friend or her brother.

If it seems as though your child is doing plenty of activities, remember Irene, our soccer goalie, whose activities weren't as active as they appeared. On page 38, we listed the sports in order—starting with the ones that are generally least intense, and proceeding to those that tend to be more intense. Baseball and softball, for example, involve more waiting around than running around, while swimming laps can be quite strenuous.

With regard to classes, taking an art or music class is better than sitting in front of the TV, but to increase the intensity of activity, see if your child would like to add one of the other classes on the list, such as martial arts or swimming. You don't have to bring it up in terms of increasing activity to help his weight. Just ask him if he'd like to do something new that's fun. If he's hesitant to go by himself, maybe he would like to take the class with a friend. It's always more fun with a buddy.

Question 7 specifically referred to weekend activities, although they also can be done during the week. And question 8 asked about household chores that are somewhat active. What you want to look at here is the intensity. The activities were listed from least active to most active.

Inactive: video games, watching TV, sitting at the computer, going to the movies

Moderately active: bowling, horseback riding, Ping-Pong, Frisbee, catch, hopscotch, hitting a tennis ball, downhill skiing, and dancing, as well as the household activities in question 8

Active: hiking, tennis, roller-skating, ice skating, bicycling, cross-country skiing, walking, and swimming

Very active: jogging, jumping rope

You can use this part of the assessment to find activities in the "moderately active" or "active" category that your child does *sometimes* and see if he would be able to do them more *often*. Or he might want to do some of the *moderate* activities a little less often, and try a new *active* pursuit. However, it's best not to do both at the same time. In other words, it may be too much to try to move up to a higher activity level, while at the same time increasing the frequency of exercise. Remember: Gradual changes are the ones that are most likely to stick.

Why Isn't Your Child More Active?

Some children will welcome the opportunity to do a new activity, while other children will resist engaging in anything physical. Here are some possible reasons why your child might not be excited about exercise.

She's not interested. Every child is different. One child will turn up her nose at ice skating, while another thinks it's cool. The most straightforward approach is to ask your child what activities she'd like to do. But don't assume that she will be able to think of every possibility. You may need to make some suggestions. After all, she can't be interested in something she's never heard about. You may also give her the opportunity to try something new—with no strings attached—to see if she likes it.

Another way to increase your child's interest in a particular activity or sport is to be enthusiastic about it yourself. Instead of saying, "I think you'd have fun if you went for a walk," try, "It's such a beautiful day, I'm going for a walk in the park, would you like to join me?"

For younger children, you will create interest in activities by buying them a new toy that requires active play: perhaps a Frisbee, a jump rope, a kite, a pair of skates, a hula hoop, or a tether ball for the backyard. Anything new is bound to generate interest, at least for a while.

Paying older children to do active chores may be an effective way to pique their interest. Washing the car, carrying groceries, raking leaves, vacuuming, and walking the dog are all somewhat active.

He doesn't feel talented in sports. No one likes to make a fool of himself. If your child isn't naturally athletic, but would like to participate in a certain sport, perhaps you could help him practice until he feels better about his abilities. If he can build his confidence in the basic skills required, he might have the courage to try playing with other children.

Another alternative is to encourage activities that don't involve competition. Anyone can walk, and learning to ride a bicycle, rollerskate, or throw a Frisbee is well within the reach of most children. The best part about noncompetitive sports is that there's no winner, so there's no loser.

She doesn't have time. If your child wants to be more active, but can't find the time, maybe you can help her with a little time management. As we've said, the best place to start is by reducing TV or computer time. However, if she doesn't spend a lot of time in front of the television, maybe she's talking on the phone or hanging out in the mall more than she thinks.

He finds exercise too uncomfortable. An overweight child, in particular, might find it uncomfortable to engage in certain activities. If he's been sedentary for quite a while, he might get out of breath walking up a hill or playing an active sport. Or he might feel okay while he's exercising, but the sore muscles that come the next day make him not want to do it again. The best way to deal with this issue is prevention. By maintaining a moderate approach to duration and intensity, your child is less likely to find the activity uncomfortable, either while he's doing it or afterwards.

She's embarrassed. If your child is embarrassed because she feels awkward doing certain physical activities, don't push her to join a class with other children. She'll feel more at ease with her family or best friend than with a bunch of strangers. Or maybe she wants to be completely alone, doing an exercise video at home.

Perhaps it's not the activity itself that bothers her, but the costume that goes with the activity. For example, if she's embarrassed to be seen in a bathing suit, don't make her swim. Find out if there's something else she'd like to do instead.

Starting an Exercise Program

If your child is ready to begin a moderate exercise program, we'd like to recommend walking, biking, or swimming. First, they're all relatively easy and they don't require much equipment or expense. They're not difficult to learn, no athletic talent is required, and there's little opportunity for failure.

Second, they're flexible enough to meet the needs of just about any child. In fact, walking, biking, and swimming are infinitely flexible when it comes to frequency, intensity, and duration. This makes them appropriate for beginners as well as more advanced exercisers. Plus, any of these activities can become sports if your child wants to pursue one of them at a higher level. They're also flexible in that they can be done alone or with others. And they are suitable for cross training: doing two, or all three, at different times of the year or on different days of the week. And they can be done indoors or outdoors, depending upon the weather and equipment available.

Finally, children tend to like walking, biking, and swimming. And adults enjoy these activities, too, so they are more likely to become lifetime healthy habits than in-line skating or field hockey.

Walking is the universal exercise. Once a child learns to walk, he never forgets how. There's no training involved. Just put one foot in front of the other. A child can start naturally with family trips to the shopping mall, walks around the zoo, and neighborhood jaunts. Walking gives a child the opportunity to socialize with his parents or with friends. Walking helps a child get in touch with the environment, whether it's in the city or in the country. Walking or hiking in parks or nature preserves can be particularly enjoyable.

If your child is interested in walking regularly, she might start with a ten-minute walk every day to begin establishing this activity as a regular habit. As she gets more comfortable, she can work up to walking a mile a day. Walking at a moderate pace, it takes about twenty minutes to go a mile. She should walk continuously, without stopping. Over time, she can increase intensity (walk faster) and duration (walk longer). Some children like to chart their progress, so you might buy your child an exercise log to keep track of her walking frequency, time, and distance.

In the next chapter, "Make Exercise Fun," we've got lots of suggestions for adding interest and entertainment value to walks with your child.

Kids and bicycles just seem to go together. Your child might consider biking more fun than walking. Even the most sedentary, television-addicted youngster will climb on a bike once in a while. Riding a bicycle can be performed without a great deal of effort, which makes it ideal for a sedentary child. But it also can be exhilarating, so if he gets started, perhaps he'll get hooked on the fun of it.

A good prescription for an inactive child who is just beginning to bike regularly is to go on an easy ride, for fifteen to twenty minutes, every other day. As he gains more confidence and endurance, he can gradually increase the frequency to every day. Next, he can begin to work on intensity and duration, as appropriate.

The only concern about riding bikes is making the activity as safe as possible. Teach your child to always wear a helmet and to ride safely around cars.

Swimming is great summer fun. Swimming is popular with children of all ages. However, swimming for exercise is different than playing around in the pool. Jumping into the pool, playing water volleyball, or diving for coins do qualify as activities, but for significant exercise benefits, your child will have to swim laps.

Swimming is particularly attractive during summer months, when it might be too hot or humid to walk or bike in the middle of the day.

The potential downside to swimming is that an overweight child may be reluctant to be seen in a bathing suit in public. But if your youngster likes the water and wants to learn to swim, we encourage you to let her.

Swimming with sufficient intensity to improve fitness and burn calories does require a certain amount of skill. So unless your child already knows how to do the crawl and breast and back strokes, lessons from a qualified instructor will be the starting point for his swimming program. Many schools and community centers offer classes for children.

The instructor can help your child figure out how long and how far she should swim. And when she is able to swim for thirty minutes without stopping, three or four times a week, she'll be working hard enough and long enough to become physically fit.

In conclusion, we would like you to keep in mind three lessons about exercise.

Exercise Lesson 1: Every little activity helps.
Exercise Lesson 2: Doing more is better.
Exercise Lesson 3: If it's not fun, your child won't do it at all.

So in the next chapter we're going to help you make exercise fun for you and your child.

20

Make Exercise Fun

Do you remember how Tom Sawyer got the neighborhood boys to whitewash the fence for him? He tricked them into thinking that he was doing them a big favor by letting them participate in something special. Now we're not suggesting that you fool your child into thinking that exercise is enjoyable. Instead, we want you to use some of Tom's creative spirit to make exercise *truly* fun for your child.

There are four variations on this theme:

1. Play up the *activity* in play.
2. Don't spoil sports.
3. Make fitness fun.
4. Promote active projects.

Parents and children have different roles and responsibilities when it comes to exercise, just as they do with food. It is the parent's responsibility to provide options for activity, while it is the child's role to choose which ones she would like to do. One child might be thrilled by competition, while another would rather participate in exercises where the goal is simply to be active and have a good time.

Another important consideration in choosing a physical activity is your child's age and skill level. Because every child is different, we haven't attempted to assign age ranges to specific activities: It's up to you and your child to determine what's fun and appropriate.

Play Up the Activity in Play

Small children don't need any motivation to exercise. They do it all the time. It's called playing. For them, play often involves seeking out opportunities to run, jump, leap, climb, spin, bounce, and scramble.

But as children grow older, their play tends to become less active. And while any kind of indoor or outdoor fun that involves moving around is better than sitting around, the more active the activity the better.

Here are some ideas for activities your child can do by himself or herself, as long as the basic equipment is available.

- *Jumping rope:* If your child is goal-oriented, she could count how many times she jumps over the rope without missing and then try to improve on her personal best. Or she could jump rope to music with a steady beat to help establish her rhythm and pace.
- *Shooting baskets:* Do you have a place for a basketball hoop on the side of your house or garage? If there's no outside location, what about Nerf basketball in the family room?
- *Dancing:* All it takes is music and a little space. It doesn't even have to disturb your peace and quiet if your child has a Walkman.
- *Tennis:* Although your child can't play a game of tennis by himself, he can practice by hitting balls against the side of the house or against the wall at the playground.
- *Hula hoops and hobby horses:* Look at the toy store for toys such as these that promote active play.

Playing with other children adds to the fun.

- *Basketball free throws:* When the player makes a basket, she gets to throw again. When she misses, the next player gets to shoot. See who can get twenty baskets first.
- *Hopscotch:* All they need is chalk and some sidewalk.
- *Tennis:* Are there tennis courts nearby? Are they convenient to get to?
- *Volleyball:* If you don't have an official volleyball net, improvise with a rope or plastic banners strung between two poles or a pair of trees.
- *Nerf paddle ball:* Using Ping-Pong or other paddles, hit a Nerf ball or balloon around among the various players. This is a good indoor activity for a rainy day.
- *Frisbee toss:* Pack a Frisbee along with the lunch when you go on a picnic.

- *Jump rope games:* Two to turn the rope, one or more to jump. Children can make up their own games and rhymes, as they jump over a single rope or do Double Dutch.
- *Dodge ball:* Remember this traditional favorite?

Some activities need a leader, such as a parent or older sibling.

- *Active story-telling:* One way to encourage movement in little children is to tell imaginary stories about animals, cartoon heroes, or storybook characters and let your child act out the stories.
- *Follow the leader:* This can be as active as you want to make it. Have the kids run, hop, skip, march, do jumping jacks, dance. Just keep them moving as you lead them around.
- *Races:* Organize some fun races in the backyard. Games that even the odds, such as potato sack races, carrying an egg on a spoon, or three-legged races are extra fun. Figure out a way for each child to win at something.

These are just a few ideas to get your creative juices flowing. But remember: There is no right way or wrong way to play. As long as no one gets hurt, try to leave it up to your child to create the rules or decide that there aren't any.

Don't Spoil Sports

Kids play sports in order to have fun. And statistics show that children are joining sports teams in record numbers. However, they also quit in record numbers when the fun is gone. Estimates are that 70 percent of children enrolled in youth sports activities will quit by the time they turn thirteen.

There are a number of reasons for this high dropout rate. Some children simply lose interest in the sport or become involved in other pursuits. Others get burned out by the relentless practice sessions and the intense competition of the games. The demands of schoolwork or social activities may also squeeze out sports. But, often the reason children give up on sports is that their parents chase the fun away.

The first mistake a parent can make is to pressure a child into playing a sport. A father who played baseball as a youngster may push his son to follow in his footsteps. Or maybe Dad wasn't able to play a sport and wants his child to have the opportunity he didn't. In either case, it's fine to expose a youngster to a variety of sports and even to encourage him to try a certain activity. However, it's up to the child to decide whether he wants to participate. Most young children want to please their parents and may end up playing a particular sport just to make their parents happy. But, in the long run, if they're not having fun themselves, they'll find some way to drop off the team.

Another way a parent can squelch a child's enthusiasm for a sport is to criticize her performance. Parents should be cheerleaders, not critics. Not only will a child start to doubt her own physical abilities, she will come to dread the sport because of the negative feelings associated with it. Instead of pointing out your child's mistakes, praise her personal achievements. Look for positive trends to comment on. Even though her team lost the game, did she block more goals than last week? Did she hit more of her tennis serves "in" than "out" during today's match?

Participation is the key for children. Studies have shown that children who participate in sports would rather play on a losing team than sit on the bench of a team that's winning. That isn't to say that children do not get a thrill from winning. Things go wrong when parents overemphasize winning and downplay the other positive features of team sports, such as team spirit, fun, and fitness. Parents don't do this intentionally. Some simply get caught up in the excitement of the games. Others forget that it's a child's team and try to apply professional standards to the mini-athletes on the field.

There's another adult who can spoil sports for your child—the team's coach. It's important to find a coach who shares your positive values. When considering an exercise program or sports team, interview the coach before you sign your child up for the program. For example, what is the coach's policy about how much and how often each child gets to play? Does she design activities to accommodate students of varying physical characteristics and ability levels? Does he emphasize sportsmanship and social skills as well as skills in catching, throwing, and batting? Does she teach the children about fitness and healthy living?

Make Fitness Fun

Perhaps your child's idea of fun has nothing to do with team sports. Instead, she may enjoy more individual pursuits that are competitive, such as tennis or swimming, or noncompetitive, such as biking, skiing, or walking. Support her participation in any physical activity she enjoys. And it doesn't have to be just one sport or activity. Variety adds fun, too.

Another way to make fitness fun is to encourage sports that are appropriate for the child's developmental level. Children develop athletic abilities at different rates. Some develop basic skills, such as catching or hitting a ball, at four or five years of age, while others aren't proficient until they're eight or nine. If a child is a late bloomer, she may not be as successful at certain sports as other children her age.

However, don't assume that he'll never be able to play these sports or do certain activities. There's a real danger in labeling your child as "not athletic" simply because he seems to lag behind others in his class. If he gets that message from you and comes to believe that he lacks athletic abilities, he may stop trying.

Unfortunately, many overweight or sedentary children put the label "not athletic" on themselves, after repeatedly being chosen last for teams or suffering insults from their peers for their performance. When they observe that they can't play as well as other children, they're likely to give up on exercise. After all, no one likes to do something they don't do well. If your child wants to learn to play better, perhaps you can help him practice basic skills. Then give him the opportunity to try the sport again, when he's feeling more confident and competent.

In order for a child to enjoy exercise, she needs to feel successful by whatever standard is meaningful to her. It may have nothing to do with winning; instead "success" could be based on individual achievement, from simply sticking with an exercise program, to increasing the duration or frequency of the exercise, to achieving a personal best. Children are much more likely to continue exercising if they can see their progress and know that their parents notice and value their efforts, too. You may want to consider ways to recognize your child for exercising regularly, such as putting up a wall calendar and placing a star or sticker on it each time your child exercises.

We've said it before, but we'll say it again—start slowly. No child is going to find exercise fun if the session involves sweating, straining, panting, or pain. Too much of a good thing is still too much. For example, let's say your child is enjoying a moderate hike in the forest and is enthusiastic when you stop for lunch midway on the route. Don't risk turning her delight into distress by choosing a more difficult path for the return trip. If she staggers to the car exhausted, chances are the next time you mention the word *hike*, she's going to take a hike in the opposite direction. You want your child to remember how it feels to complete a good hike, challenged but comfortable.

Another way to make fitness fun is to add adventure to activity. If you live or vacation near a river, lake, or bay, you might try kayaking or canoeing. There are classes offered for children and adults at many recreational areas. Or if the water is warm, how about snorkeling?

Another option is to send your child to sports camp if he has the desire. There are a multitude of camps around the country that provide children with focused instruction in such sports as baseball, basketball, and tennis. During the one to four weeks a child spends at camp, he can greatly enhance his skills. And with those new skills comes greater self-confidence and, perhaps, a new incentive to keep exercising.

Closer to home, maybe there are aerobics classes designed for youngsters. It's a noncompetitive form of exercise that helps improve coordination and stamina. Martial arts classes are also popular with many children, both boys and girls.

Walking is still the easiest and most versatile of all exercises. And while in its purest form, it may not be a child's idea of fun, it doesn't take much to turn it into a pleasant pastime.

- Buy your child a portable music player so she can listen to the radio or favorite tunes while she walks. Music that's fast-paced can help speed up the pace of walking.
- Tell stories while you walk. You tell the first one, and then it's your child's turn to make one up. Keep alternating. You'll be amazed at how the time flies.
- Get your child a camera to take photographs on family walks. Inexpensive, single-use cameras might be good for younger children.

- To keep your child busy on a city walk, have him find all the letters in the alphabet—in the proper sequence—by looking at street signs, stores, license plates, buses, billboards, etc.
- When you go for a hike or walk at the beach or in the woods, take along a plastic bag for your child to collect treasures, such as rocks, shells, leaves, or pine cones. When you get home, she can put some of them into a Walk Book. Depending on her age, you can encourage or help your child label the pages with the date, where you walked, who went, and what your child saw. Or the items collected could be used for art projects.
- Organize a "mental" scavenger hunt. Prior to the walk, make up a list of items that your child could find on the route. The object isn't to actually collect the items, but rather to call them out and mark them off the list as he spots them. During a walk in the city, he could look for such things as a parked truck, a laundromat, a penny on the ground, a neon sign, and a toy store. In the woods, the items could be a squirrel, a particular kind of wild flower, a waterfall, a bird's nest, and a spider web.
- Let your child play "navigator." Plan out a route for her and a friend to follow through the neighborhood. You can either draw a map that graphically shows where to go, or write down detailed descriptions of the route. Make it interesting and as challenging to follow as appropriate for the children. The trail can take them to a surprise destination or it can simply follow a course that leads them back home.

Promote Active Projects

Some children get great satisfaction out of doing projects that have tangible results. It might be a project to build or create something, or one that allows them to earn a little spending money. Or it could be a community service project where the reward comes from doing something that helps others. In any case, perhaps you can steer your child toward projects that not only provide one of these benefits, but offer some exercise value as well.

For example, a creative project that involves a moderate amount of exercise is planting and taking care of vegetables or flowers in the garden. Helping Mom or Dad prepare the soil, dig holes, and plant the plants can be fairly active. And staying involved as the plants grow—watering, weeding, and trimming—can give a child a sense of accomplishment. Plus, there's an added benefit if you plant vegetables. Your child will be more likely to eat the vegetables he helped grow than the ones that come from the supermarket.

Community service projects can benefit one person or many. For example, a number of nonprofit organizations have walk-a-thons or bike-a-thons as fund-raisers. Perhaps your child would enjoy collecting pledges for participating in one of these events. Depending upon the length of the course, she may have to do a little advance "training" to be able to go the distance.

Another way to help the community and get some exercise at the same time is to help clean up a local beach. Sometimes environmental groups organize such outings. But you don't have to wait for a special day. The next time you go to the beach, take along garbage bags and disposable rubber gloves. You can turn it into a game if you bring along a timer, too. See who can collect the most litter in a set period of time. At day's end, recycle the bottles and cans and dump the nonrecyclables in the nearest trash receptacle.

For community service on a more personal level, your child might feel good about helping an elderly or disabled neighbor who is unable to do physically demanding chores. Your child could wash the car, carry groceries, and sweep the walkway or porch on a regular basis, as well as shovel snow in the winter or rake leaves in the fall.

Your child could do these same kinds of chores around your house, too, but you'll probably need to provide some monetary motivation or other kind of tangible reward. Although, if you're as creative as Tom Sawyer, perhaps you can think of a way to turn such active projects into playful activities.

21

Fitness for the Whole Family

EVERY FAMILY HAS A CULTURE: a set of habits, practices, and customs that have been established over time and have come to be accepted as "the way we do things." Elements of a family's culture can range from religious practices to vacation preferences; from what kind of music they listen to in the car to whether they eat Thanksgiving dinner at home or go to Grandma's for the day. Another element of a family's culture is its choice of leisure activities.

If you take a look back at the Family Favorites Chart on page 41, you'll get a picture of your family's culture with regard to activities. Are most of your favorites and your child's in the top half of the chart, activities like watching television and going to the movies? Perhaps you have more favorites in the bottom half of the chart than your child does: You enjoy hiking and working out at the gym, while your youngster would rather talk on the telephone or play video games. Or it could be that your whole family enjoys active leisure pursuits, but you just don't make time for them in your schedule. In any case, planning for more fun physical activities can benefit the whole family, especially your chubby child.

And planning is what it will take, because increasing activity doesn't just happen. You'll have to make a conscious effort to think of ways to add exercise to current activities and to replace certain sedentary habits with more active ones. The effort required might be substantial, but the ultimate payoff will be more than worth it. If you can find activities that your family enjoys and you all do them often enough, over time you will establish new, healthy habits that will become part of your family culture.

Children Learn Best by Example

Children often use their parents as the inspiration for new games to play. What little boy hasn't asked his father if he can shave some imaginary whiskers off his beardless chin? And what little girl hasn't dressed up in her mother's clothes and preened in front of the mirror, teetering on a pair of oversized pumps? Wouldn't it be great if your child wanted to follow in your footsteps—literally—by walking, jogging, or engaging in some other form of exercise she sees you doing?

But what if your child's role models are currently sedentary ones? Then it's time for you and your spouse to get off the couch and encourage your child to follow. Just the fact that you're making the effort to be more active may serve as an inspiration to your child. Or perhaps you and your child can support each other by exercising together.

If you currently exercise and your child isn't following your example, give some thought to why that might be. Do you exercise reluctantly or talk more about how hard your workouts are than how good they make you feel? Perhaps your child thinks that exercise is too uncomfortable to want to try it herself.

If it's really not as bad as you make out, and you think your child would enjoy your preferred form of exercise, start talking more positively about it and then invite him to join you sometime. But be prepared to tone down or otherwise modify your program so that it's an appropriate start for your child. And if your usual activity is a game, such as tennis or racquetball, remember that children can't compete on an adult level. Give your child a scoring advantage to even the odds so that he can win sometimes. After all, no one wants to keep playing a game they always lose.

If you want to keep your current routine, but it's not suitable for your child, consider adopting some activities that you and your child can do together in addition to your own personal workout.

Role modeling a good attitude is important, too. So when you do exercise together, don't groan or complain. And resist the temptation to look at your watch every five minutes to see when you'll be finished. You want your child to get the message that physical activity is a pleasure, not a chore.

And role modeling isn't confined to just traditional exercises. You also can role model increasing activity in general. For example, take the stairs instead of the elevator, and seek out opportunities to walk places instead of driving.

Family Support for Your Child

Changing a habit is no easy task. Mark Twain captured this sentiment perfectly when he said, "Habit is habit and not to be flung out of the window by any man, but coaxed downstairs a step at a time." Likewise, try to increase your family's activity level one step at a time. So in addition to modeling active behavior, it's important for you to support your child's attempts at being more active.

For example, give positive reinforcement to any active behavior your child demonstrates, and refrain from negative comments. Don't push your child, but if she has started to do some kind of exercise, verbalize your support and encouragement. And on days when her motivation flags, you can *physically* demonstrate your support by offering to exercise with her.

Also, you may have to make some personal sacrifices in order to help your child be more active. For example, you might have to give up one of your own activities in order to fit in exercising with your child or to support him when he plays team sports. And if the family activity your child enjoys isn't your personal favorite, be a good sport anyway. You may find yourself liking it more than you thought you would.

Plan Family Outings That Include Exercise

Like most parents, you probably wish you could spend more quality time with your child. "If only there were more hours in the day," you lament. You might be surprised at how many extra hours you could find if you cut down on family television viewing. Although watching TV together is a family activity, it hardly counts as quality time, especially when the conversation consists of "Pass the chips" and "Shshsh, I'm trying to watch the program."

One strategy for breaking the ties that bind your family to the television set is to use your VCR to tape programs while you're not home. If you don't know how, ask your child or read the owner's manual. With this new skill, you can plan an active family outing on a Saturday afternoon without having to miss the ball game. And when you come home, you'll be able to watch the game in less time than if you had watched it "live" because you can fast-forward through the commercials.

In contrast to television time, family activity time offers a wonderful opportunity for talking with your child and, perhaps more important, for really listening to her. Your child's initial resistance to getting off the couch will probably be overcome by the realization that she will have your undivided time and attention. You can have some great conversations with your child when you don't have to compete with the television or telephone.

When planning a family outing, don't be surprised if various members of the family have trouble agreeing on the best way to have fun. Flexibility is the key, but remember that your goal is to try to increase your overweight child's activity level. So try to plan something that she will enjoy.

With just one child, this shouldn't be too difficult, but with two or three, you will have to be resourceful. Try to find at least one activity that the whole family can enjoy together. If a particular activity doesn't suit your family, go on to something else. And keep trying new activities to expand the family's fitness repertoire.

It probably won't be a struggle to get a young child to go along with the family activity agenda, but when children grow older, they are more apt to be set in their sedentary ways. Or, if they're teenagers, they won't be wild about spending time with their parents under any circumstances. Still, letting your child suggest activities and bring a friend along may make a family activity more acceptable.

Another strategy to increase participation is to tailor the activity so it's suitable for the different skill levels of your children. For example, on a bike ride, Dad may need to pedal at a slower pace with your five-year-old, while Mom goes on ahead with your twelve-year-old.

Maybe you can get everyone involved if you start a Future Family Activities List. Hang it on the refrigerator where any family member can add to it. The only rule is that the suggestions have to be "active." Then use the list to spark ideas for weekend outings. Just be sure that each family member gets his or her first choice some of the time.

Here are some ideas to get your list started. And don't be put off because you don't know how to do a particular sport. Seize the opportunity to learn a new activity along with your child. That's part of the fun and it also enhances family togetherness.

- Bicycling
- Walking
- In-line skating
- Ice-skating
- Swimming
- Bowling
- Skiing
- Tennis
- Hiking

Although a number of these activities are particularly suited to weekends, we urge you to add family fitness activities to your weekday schedule, too. Walking, for example, can work well after dinner. You can walk around your neighborhood or drive to a nearby location for a pleasant change of pace. In the summer, when it stays light later, you can even go to the beach or to the park.

Another way to incorporate fitness into your family is to join a health club that has programs for both adults and children. We're not talking about a club that just has a baby-sitting service. Look for one that has children's exercise classes. Some clubs offer movement, dancing, and circuit training as well as step aerobics for youngsters. Your child will feel so grown up when she tells her friends that she's going to the gym with Mom or Dad.

And once you've added exercise to your family's lifestyle, don't revert back to your sedentary ways when you go on vacation. Plan vacations that provide ample opportunity for exercise, whether it's swimming and river rafting in the summer, or skiing and snowshoeing in the winter. Again, the activities don't have to be sports. You could take a trip that includes walking tours of interesting cities or hikes in the country.

Take a Family Hike

Hiking offers many advantages, on vacation or anytime during the year: It doesn't require special equipment (just an appropriate pair of shoes); it can be adapted to any fitness level; it promotes family inter-action; it offers a change of scenery; and it can be fun enough to become a lifelong healthy habit.

If you've never planned a family hike, here are some things to consider. In fact, you can adapt many of these principles to suit other outdoor family activities.

- Go to your local bookstore or library for a guide to hiking trails in your area.
- Choose a route that is appropriate for all members of the family. If you're trying to decide between two hikes, pick the easier one.
- Choose a route that's suitable for the season and the weather on the day of your hike. Don't choose a shadeless trail in the middle of summer or a windswept beach in the middle of winter.
- Ask your child if he would like to bring a friend along for company.
- Be sure your child has appropriate clothing. Layers are best so she can take a sweater off or put a jacket on as needed to be comfortable.
- If the adults are wearing back packs or fanny packs, get a small one for your child and let him carry something in it so he feels like an "official" hiker.
- Set a realistic pace. Little legs can't walk as fast as big ones. Besides, children may want to slow down from time to time to investigate interesting items along the trail.
- Stop at regular intervals. Children on the hike may need to rest more often than the adults.
- Bring along plenty of water and healthy snacks or lunch.
- Provide encouragement to your child by telling her what a ter-rific hiker she is.
- Set a positive example for your youngster by being a good sport. Even if you're tired on the way back, keep smiling.
- Look at page 203 to refresh your memory about ways to make walking more fun. Some of these suggestions could enhance a family hike, too.

Although your motivation for increasing family fitness activities is to help your chubby child, you're going to get a lot out of it, too. Exercise can energize you when you're tired, and you'll feel better the more fit you become.

Keep in mind that the activities you and your family choose have to be compatible with your lifestyle, or they won't have a chance of becoming part of the family culture. However, if you're successful, you'll be giving your child a valuable legacy: the lifelong image of herself as an active person, not a couch potato.

PART V

Facilitate Change

22

Align Your Attitudes to Facilitate Change

WE ALL HAVE ATTITUDES. The trouble is that they're usually invisible. Most of the time, you don't even realize they're there, even though they are influencing every comment you make and every action you take. Only when you come face-to-face with your attitudes can you begin to change the ones that may be getting in the way of your being able to help your child.

We don't know which attitudes you have about food, exercise, being overweight, or making lifestyle changes. What we do know is that certain attitudes about these subjects will assist in your efforts to help your overweight child, while others are more likely to sabotage them. For example, if you believe that your youngster shouldn't have to finish everything on his plate, he's less likely to become a member of the Clean-Plate Club. Or if your opinion of exercise is that it's too much trouble, you probably won't encourage your child to be more active. And without your participation and support, your child isn't likely to turn off the television and get off the couch.

What Are Your Attitudes?

Attitudes remain invisible unless we focus our attention on them. A good way to start is to do a personal attitude check. Do you agree or disagree with the following statements?

1. In order to lose weight, you have to follow a strict diet.
2. In order to lose weight, you can't eat your favorite foods.

3. In order to lose weight, you have to go hungry.
4. Eating snacks between meals makes you gain weight.
5. In order to lose weight, you have to exercise strenuously.
6. Exercise isn't important for weight loss; it's the food that matters.
7. Exercise makes you eat more.
8. A parent needs to get mad when an overweight child eats something "fattening."
9. A parent needs to control how much a child eats.
10. Withholding food is an effective punishment for misbehavior.
11. Giving food treats is a good way to reward children for desirable behavior.
12. An overweight child should be able to exert self-control and not eat candy, even when others are.
13. Children should eat whatever their parents put on their plates.
14. When it comes to food and exercise, children should do what their parents say, not necessarily what they do.
15. Children become overweight because they eat too much.
16. Overweight people are different from normal weight people.
17. It's helpful to repeatedly remind an overweight child about her eating behaviors.
18. You shouldn't spend money on new clothes until you've lost weight.
19. The proper body shape for a girl is tall and thin.
20. The proper body shape for a boy is tall and muscular.

We hope that you disagreed with most, if not all, of the statements listed. We have discussed many of these issues in earlier chapters, so you probably have already incorporated some of this new knowledge into your way of thinking, shifting your attitudes toward more positive approaches to weight control.

However, consider the statements you *agreed* with. These are the ones that are most likely to sabotage your attempts to help your child lose weight the healthy way. Where might these attitudes have come from? Often they're passed on from one generation to the next. For example, if you withhold food as a punishment or use food treats as a reward, your parents may have done the same thing with you.

Sometimes we adopt attitudes that are the opposite of our parents' values. Individuals who grew up with parents who were overly strict about food—forbidding eating between meals or restricting second helpings—may appropriately decide to never deprive their own children of food. However, instead of a comfortable, moderate approach, their attitude may cause them to go too far, becoming overly lenient with regard to food and providing no limits or guidance for their children about healthy eating behaviors.

When considering the origin of attitudes, we cannot overlook some of the most potent influences: what we see on television, hear on the radio, and read in magazines and newspapers. Television alone is filled with news programs, talk shows, sitcoms, and soap operas that send subtle, and not-so-subtle, messages about food, exercise, weight, and body shape. While some promote health, many do not. This includes one of the most pervasive themes: that fat is bad and thin is good—the thinner the better. These kinds of messages not only influence adults, they also have a profound effect on our children.

How can you work on changing a counterproductive attitude once you recognize you have it? Some attitudes can be realigned simply by gaining the appropriate knowledge to make the shift. For example, maybe you thought that forbidding between-meal snacks was an appropriate way to help your child with his weight. But based on information we have presented in this book, you now realize that healthy snacks can help prevent a child from overeating at meals. You may not need any more input in order to begin providing appropriate snacks.

On the other hand, it takes more than knowledge to dislodge a firmly rooted attitude. Sometimes reflecting on its possible origin can be useful. If you can figure out where your opinion originated, maybe you'll see that it came from an unreliable source or is based on an isolated incident or false premise. Or perhaps it will just help you to understand your thinking and be open to changing it.

Sometimes the advice and counsel of a friend or family member can help you gain perspective on your attitudes. Perhaps by talking to someone you trust, you can begin to see things differently.

We would like to make an important point about attitudes. They don't just come in black and white. They come in all shades of gray.

You don't have to embrace a particular attitude 100 percent in order for it to help you facilitate the changes you want to make. Just try to recognize and lighten up some of your negative attitudes.

Realigning Your Attitudes About Change

Many of the themes we've presented throughout the book have related to attitudes about change. In case you didn't think of them as attitudes, we'll take a moment to recap some of the more significant ones. Our focus here isn't on change for the sake of change, but rather on change strategies that will result in long-term, healthy weight control for your child.

Moderate changes are most effective. It is a common assumption that if a little of something is good, a lot must be better. While this may be true of fame and fortune, when it comes to modifying behaviors, moderate changes work better than excessive ones. Children rebel against radical changes and parents burn out trying to implement them. That's why extreme measures don't work in the long run. No one can keep doing them.

Imagine what would happen if you suddenly switched every possible food in your kitchen to a fat-free version. But why cause a riot, when a moderate approach to choosing lower-fat products works much better? It's easier to slip in a low-fat salad dressing here and a fat-free cracker there. And, in fact, moderation is all that's needed to help your child with her weight. Changes that are comfortable enough to be repeated again and again form the foundation of long-term success.

Change has to be gradual to be successful. Changes need to be made slowly because it takes time to learn new habits. That's because learning a new behavior *well* takes practice, just like learning to ride a bicycle. And you wouldn't expect your child to go directly from riding a tricycle to mastering a mountain bike. It would be just as disastrous to try to get your child to give up potato chips "cold turkey." But using the "training wheel" technique, you could try cutting down on how often she has chips and how many she eats, then switch to lower-fat ones and, eventually, maybe even to chips that are baked, not fried. And just as we never forget how to ride a bicycle, if a child learns a new healthy eating behavior and practices it over time, it has a good chance of becoming a lifelong habit.

Changes have to be acceptable to your child and meet his or her needs. If a change is acceptable to a child, he'll try it; and if it meets his needs, he'll keep doing it. Sometimes you can nudge your child to get him to try something new and he'll end up liking it. But if you try to force a change that isn't a good fit, it won't last. For example, if you push your child into playing baseball and make him continue even if he resists, it may result not only in his disliking baseball, but in a general aversion to all sports. A better approach would be to help your child find an activity he thinks he would enjoy and let him try it out to see if it's right for him.

Changes in habits have to be for the whole family. Treating your child differently from the rest of the family is not fair or effective. If you single your chubby child out for unusual treatment, she may get the message that there's something wrong with her or that she's being punished for being overweight. For example, denying your child a rich dessert, while everyone else gets to eat it, is not only unfair, it will make her crave desserts even more. Just because your child may have some extra weight, there is no reason to deprive her of pleasures the rest of the family is able to enjoy. A more effective and even-handed approach would be to offer more nutritious, lower-calorie desserts for the whole family. And when you do serve a high-calorie dessert as a treat, everyone should be allowed to indulge—but maybe in healthier portions.

Changes have to be compatible with your family's lifestyle. Although the focus of your efforts is your overweight child, many of the changes you're going to make will affect the whole family. Other family members are likely to resent changes that affect their lives in a negative way. And, worse for your child, they may come to resent him, too. So it's important to make sure that your strategies fit your family's lifestyle. For example, if eating breakfast in a special restaurant is a Sunday morning ritual, don't stop going out for breakfast. Instead, help your child to order more appropriately by role modeling and making some helpful suggestions. Or if this is the only meal you eat out all week, let everyone enjoy their favorites.

Support is the foundation for all change. Your child won't be able to make positive changes in eating and exercise without your support. It's that simple. Support will help give your child the courage to try new things, such as a new sport or activity. And your encouragement over time will help her sustain the positive changes she makes. But support isn't control. Although you can support your child's weight-loss efforts by making sure there are plenty of nutritious low-fat snacks in the house, you can't control what your child puts in her mouth.

Adjusting Your Attitudes About Weight

Now we would like to introduce some attitudes about weight and weight loss. Accepting these attitudes is essential to helping your child lose weight the healthy way.

Weight loss has to be gradual. Moderate, gradual changes will result in moderate, gradual weight loss. And that's the best kind. Not only is rapid, large weight loss potentially dangerous for your child, it's an indication that your strategies are too extreme. Besides, weight that's lost too fast is more likely to be regained even faster.

Every child is different in the way he or she loses weight. This is more of a fact than an attitude, but you'll need to accept the fact and accept the way your child loses weight. It may be that your child won't end up losing any weight at all. In this case, try to help yourself see that helping your youngster develop good eating and exercise habits that will allow him to *maintain* his weight as he grows is a successful outcome.

The bottom line is that it's important to keep your focus on healthy food and fitness behaviors—not on the scale. Besides, if you're helping your child make positive changes, the scale will take care of itself. However, if you have unrealistic expectations about your child's weight loss and try to push her to live up to them, the result will be failure. In chapter 26, we'll help you set some realistic goals for yourself and your child.

Your child's body shape is greatly influenced by genetics. Your child may be able to lose weight, but his basic shape isn't going to change dramatically. The biggest change in body shape will come with puberty. But if your child is short and stocky just like his father, and his uncle, and his grandfather, he's not likely to end up looking like a basketball player or a jockey.

So if you have some image fixed in your mind of the "perfect" body for your child, you had better give it up. Because if you send your child the message that you want her to look a certain way, she may try in vain to overcome her genetics by exercising excessively or trying to adhere to an overly strict diet.

And even if *you* don't have unrealistic expectations about your child's body shape, *she* might. In that case, you'll have to try, as best you can, to counteract the messages she's getting from her friends and through the media. One way to do this is to comment on the fact that overly thin or overly muscular bodies can only be achieved by a small percentage of people whose genes allow them to develop these kinds of bodies.

Your child is not a bad person if he or she is overweight. Let your child know that he is worthy and lovable, no matter what he weighs. His being a good person shouldn't be dependent on his size or weight. However, if you have the attitude that your youngster is overweight because he has no willpower, you may view his being overweight as a character flaw. This kind of attitude will make you feel frustrated and angry that your child is overweight and prevent you from relating to him in a healthy way. It also can make your child feel guilty about his weight or even think that you don't love him. And since many children eat to comfort themselves when they are upset or unhappy, these kinds of painful feelings are likely to make things worse.

So if you have trouble with the fact that your child is overweight, try not to focus on it. Instead, focus on your youngster's attributes that you are genuinely pleased with, such as his intelligence, sense of humor, or talent for playing the guitar. Let him know how proud you are of him for these special qualities.

Your child's circumstances aren't exactly like yours. Even if you have a weight problem, it's important to recognize that your problems aren't the same as your child's. And if you have successfully controlled your weight, you can't assume that your solutions will work for your child. But just because she's different from you doesn't mean you can't help her. First, try to understand her particular problem areas: whether it's controlling volume at a meal, liking only high-fat foods, or being reluctant to exercise. Then help her discover solutions that are right for her. Some of your own personal strategies may be effective for your child, but you'll also need to brainstorm some new ones. Remember, what's easy for you may be difficult for her. After all, you've had a lot more time to get to know how your body works. Your child is just learning.

And what if you're naturally thin? It may be particularly difficult for you to identify with your child's weight problem, but it shouldn't keep you from being supportive. By reading this book, you've taken the first step in trying to gain knowledge and understanding. The next step is to help your child adopt some of the behaviors we've outlined, as well as to teach her some of the healthy habits that come naturally to you.

Your child's overweight is nobody's "fault." That's right. It's not your fault and it's not his fault. It is simply the result of the way heredity, food, and fitness interact. Blaming uses up a lot of energy and sidetracks you from the real issues. When you can accept that your child's weight doesn't have to be blamed on anybody, you can begin to approach it as you would any other problem related to your child. That is, you can start working on positive solutions, without the distractions of judgment or blame.

It's more important to raise a healthy child than a thin one. While attempting to help your child with her weight, it's important to keep this attitude in mind. It reminds us of the Hippocratic Oath that doctors take, pledging to take actions they believe are "for the good" of their patients and to "do no harm."

Whatever strategies you try to implement for the good of your child, you must evaluate them as best you can to feel comfortable that they will do no harm, physically or emotionally. That's why we keep stressing the importance of making changes that are modest and gradual. If progress seems slow, you may have to remind yourself that you are doing what is reasonable and healthy for your child. Because if you get impatient or adamant about your child's achieving a certain weight level, you're liable to intensify your efforts and risk doing harm to your child.

Facilitate Change

Working on changing attitudes and habits is going to take time. Just remember, you're not a bad person if your attitudes aren't in perfect alignment. And you're not a failure if you can't realign them all right away. That shouldn't keep you from starting to make some changes now that will help your child lose weight the healthy way.

The first step is to make a commitment to begin changing the things you can change. As we have seen, these include some family eating behaviors, some family exercise habits, and some of your parenting techniques. Changing enough of the right things will be enough to help your child.

23

How to Talk
With Your Child

How *not* to talk to your child:

You'd be so pretty if you just lost some weight.
Do you really think you should eat that?
You can't have any dessert, you're on a diet.
*If you just had some willpower, you wouldn't have a weight
    problem.*
You're too heavy to wear a dress like that.

It's easy to come up with a list of insensitive remarks you *wouldn't*
want to make to your overweight child, but figuring out compassion-
ate ways to talk with your child about her weight is not so simple.

Should You Talk With Your Child About Her Weight?

Unless it is already an open topic of discussion, you will need to consider whether you should bring up the subject of weight with your
child. Recognizing that every child is different, here are some general
guidelines to help you decide if and when it might be an appropriate
topic to discuss.

Yes, you should talk with your child under certain circumstances.

- If the doctor tells you that your child's weight is posing a health
  risk, you will need to talk with your child, as you would if he
  had any kind of health problem. A physician will be particularly

concerned if your family has a history of heart disease or diabetes, because obesity plays a negative role in both of these life-
threatening illnesses. If the doctor talks to you privately about
your child's weight, it's your responsibility to share the doctor's
concerns with your child in a manner that is appropriate for his
age and temperament. If you think the message would be
accepted better, you could ask the doctor to discuss the issue
with you and your child together.

- If your child comes to you concerned about her weight, seize
the opportunity for a meaningful discussion. It's important to
take time to talk with her at the moment she expresses concern,
because she may not be in the mood tomorrow—and by next
week she could be more worried about her math test. Since you
have no way of predicting when your child is going to confide
in you, try to be prepared for the conversation. Think in advance
not only about how you might respond to her comments and
questions, but how to make a couple of important points of your
own. Among the messages you should try to convey are that
you love her no matter what she weighs and that you can help
her with her weight if she wants you to. You don't have to go
into detail in this first conversation. Just coming to an agreement
to work on this together will be a major accomplishment.

- If your child says he's being teased about his weight by his classmates, try to get him to talk about it and to elaborate on his
feelings about being teased. Attempt to find out what kind of
help he wants from you: Help in losing weight so he won't be a
target for teasing; help ignoring the hurtful comments; or help
asserting himself so that he won't be teased, even though he
may be overweight. For more details about how to help your
child if he's being teased, see chapter 24.

- If your child has put herself on a diet of her own creation, especially if it's too strict or ignores nutrition, it's your responsibility
to talk with her. This kind of dieting behavior could be a pass-
ing phase or it could be the early signs of an eating disorder.
Only by talking with your child will you be able to get an idea
of how serious the situation is. Calmly explain to her the risks of
crash dieting and assure her that you will help her lose weight
the healthy way.

It's better not to talk with your child about his weight when certain conditions exist.

- If your child has never brought up the subject of his weight and his overweight is not excessive, we recommend that you keep your thoughts to yourself. If his weight doesn't bother him, why risk making him self-conscious about it? However, he may be telling you in subtle ways that he is concerned and would like your help.
- If you're not able to devote the time and energy right now to help your child with her weight, we suggest that you don't discuss it. If you're not yet ready to put in the full effort required, just do the subtle things that you can easily manage.
- If your child is five or younger, there is seldom any reason to discuss her weight with her. Unless your small child starts the conversation, it's best not to bring it up. Instead of talking, just start doing. Most young children won't notice or dispute gradual changes you make in family eating and exercise habits. Your child will be likely to go along with the new program—as long as it's not too radical.

Maybe you should talk to your child and maybe you shouldn't.

- It's extremely unlikely that your youngster is going to come right out and say, "Hey Mom, will you help me lose weight in a healthy, sensible way?" So you're going to have to listen between the lines to get an idea of whether it's just you who is concerned or if both of you are worried about her weight. Your child may be in denial about her weight problem. Or maybe she's not verbalizing her anxiety, but inwardly she's hurting and wants help. Depending upon the age of your child, some things you may hear that indicate a concern about weight include:

  "Does this skirt make me look fat?"
  "I can't eat that. I'm on a diet."
  "Do I look like I've gained weight?"
  "This is the last time I'm ever going to eat pizza!"
  "Mom, you shrunk my jeans again."

Some other telltale signs are:

> not wanting to wear shorts or a bathing suit in public
> not wanting to go shopping for clothes
> not eating, or eating very sparingly, at parties or family
> gatherings
> not wanting to take her coat off at social functions

These kinds of words and actions will give you a clue that your child is upset about his size and may also serve as an opportunity to broach the subject. For example, when he says, "This is the last time I'm ever going to eat pizza," it's the perfect time to ask, "Why?" Your child might be able to say at that point that he feels fat and wants to lose weight. Once the door is open, explore ways you can help.

- If your child has recently gained weight, but hasn't mentioned it, you may be able to initiate a conversation based on your observation. But you will have to consider the possible merits and potential pitfalls of launching into such a discussion. First, think about the timing of the weight gain. If it's likely that he's put on a little weight in advance of a growth spurt, maybe you should hold off on the conversation for a while. And if you suspect that the recent weight gain is the result of a personal problem or family crisis, it would be more helpful to try to encourage him to talk about the possible root problem, rather than the symptom (the weight gain). However, if neither of these conditions seems to fit your child's situation, then you may want to initiate a calm, sensitive conversation about his weight. You might say that you've noticed that he's gained a bit of weight recently and ask him if he has any thoughts or concerns about this.
- Even if your child hasn't recently gained weight, you may still be able to bring up the subject of weight in a nonthreatening way. Perhaps you can start by asking your child an open-ended question about whether he has any thoughts or feelings about his weight. However, resist launching into the discussion just because you're feeling the need. Instead, bring up the subject at a time when your child is in the best frame of mind to be receptive and most likely to share his true feelings with you. This

might be in the car or on a walk, wherever he tends to be most relaxed. And don't expect to cover the entire subject in one session—talking about such a complex issue is more effective when done in stages.

In these three "maybe" cases, if your child doesn't want to talk about her weight, don't push. Or, if while you're talking about her weight, your child gets anxious or upset, back off. Wait for a better time and try again. Or, you can simply say, "Whenever you feel like talking about it, I'm here to help you. Just let me know."

If you decide that it's best *not* to talk to your child about his weight, there are still things you can say and do that will help him. Start initiating subtle changes in food and fitness habits, as we've suggested. And when you talk about these changes, speak in generalities. If you must comment, instead of saying, "I'm buying pretzels now because Adam shouldn't eat potato chips," say something like, "It's better for our family to eat healthier snacks."

Should You Talk With Your Child About This Book?

Back in chapter 1, we suggested that you read the entire book before deciding whether to involve your child actively in the suggestions and strategies we presented. Now that you're almost through reading, we would like to bring this subject up again.

Talking with your child about her weight or helping her with weight-loss strategies are separate issues from whether or not to mention this book to her. You'll have to ask yourself whether sharing parts of this book would help or hinder your child's weight-control efforts.

It might be helpful in a variety of situations. For example, your youngster may view your purchasing and reading a book as evidence that you really care about helping her. Or the information in the book may bolster your credibility with your child. In other words, it may be effective to say, "Don't just take my word for it—it says in this book that walking every day can help control your weight." There are times when a book by professionals may have more clout than you do.

On the other hand, the same youngster who discounts what you say may also discount the information in a book you picked out. And you probably wouldn't want to mention our book to a sensitive child who is in denial about his weight. The fact that you've purchased a book may make him feel he has a more serious problem than he thinks he has. Or trying to follow recommendations that come from a book may feel like too much pressure to your child. It may be more helpful simply to use the suggestions and not mention the source.

Even if you decide that it would be helpful to let your child know about the book, it's not appropriate to let most children read it. Since we've written the book specifically for parents, it's up to you to interpret selected information in a way that is suited to your child's individual needs. If she's old enough, you might carefully choose a few pages or a chapter to read together. Or a very independent teenager may get more out of the book by reading it herself.

Talking With Your Two- to Five-Year-Old

As we said, it's not appropriate to directly discuss issues of weight with a two- to five-year-old. However, you can take advantage of your preschooler's willingness to please his parents and his pride at doing "grown-up" things to teach him about healthy lifestyle habits. Emphasize the positive, such as, "Drinking milk helps you grow up big and strong like Daddy," or "Wouldn't it be fun to go for a walk with the big kids?"

But perhaps the easiest approach with preschoolers is to just slowly and subtly start making changes in the food you bring into the house and the kinds of activities you do as a family. Chances are your child will simply accept these changes as part of the family agenda. If, however, your child questions some new practice, answer her question as directly as you can and with just enough information to respond to the query. For example, in response to, "Why are we having fruit for dessert?" you can reply, "I'm buying more fruit now because it's healthy for our family." Don't mention anything having to do with your child or her weight.

Preschoolers especially need limits, so you will have to establish acceptable behavior with regard to such issues as how much candy is allowed, when sweets can be eaten, how many snacks are appropriate, and how close to dinner your child can eat. When you set these limits, do so in a firm manner, calmly explaining that your decisions are based on doing what's healthy for your child. Small children also need to start learning how to make choices for themselves. For example, let your child choose among grapes, an apple, or melon with her sandwich.

Talking With Your Six- to Twelve-Year-Old

Children in the middle years are like sponges, absorbing facts faster and in greater quantities than at any other time in life. Learning new information and putting that knowledge into action is what children six to twelve thrive on. This makes it the perfect time to teach your child concrete facts about nutrition, exercise, and other aspects of a healthy lifestyle that will help him grow up fit.

Gaining confidence through accomplishment is another feature of middle childhood. Therefore, if your child wants to work on her weight, it's vital that you talk to her about setting realistic goals. You may need to help her accept goals that are incremental and attainable, and then support her successful achievement of them. For example, if her preliminary goal is to take a walk three times a week, don't just leave it up to her to do it on her own, offer to walk with her. That way she's more likely to achieve this goal and feel more confident in tackling the next one.

Although parental support is vital, your child won't feel a true sense of accomplishment if you do everything for him. As with children of all ages, middle-age children need a balance between structure and freedom of choice. Younger children need more structure and less freedom of choice; teenagers need less structure and a lot more freedom of choice. But finding the appropriate balance for children in between is even trickier. You'll need to use your parental intuition to sense when to let go and when to encourage. And, as much as possible, be supportive of your child's activities and praise his positive behaviors.

If your child is working on her weight, it's especially important to help her when she slips up. So when she's upset with herself for eating too many cookies, help her to put it into perspective so she doesn't feel like a failure. You can say something like, "Don't worry about it," and remind her, "It takes time to change habits. You're used to having as many cookies as you want after school, so it will take a while to feel satisfied with only a couple."

Talking With Your Teenager

With one foot in childhood and the other in adulthood, teenagers stroll, saunter, and stagger through adolescence. A teenager's primary job is growing up, a process that involves experimenting with independence. So it's appropriate that they exercise their independence when making decisions about food. However, while practicing the skills they will use as adults, their behavior often looks like that of a child indulging in every imagined sweet or treat.

One of the factors that distinguishes adolescents from children is that they have easier access to buying food. And, as you may have noticed, their cuisine of choice is often fast-food. But since they're concerned about their bodies and how they look, they may try to counteract the burger and fries with crash dieting. Extreme, rapid weight loss is unhealthy for anybody, but it is especially dangerous for teenagers. The teen years are the last chance they have for optimal growth.

So the job of parents is to try to instill in teens the healthy eating habits that will form the foundation for the rest of their lives. It's also the last chance you have to help them stabilize their weight or shed a few pounds before the growth spurt of puberty hits.

However, the changing relationship between adolescents and their parents can make this job a touchy one. Face it, you can't abandon them and you can't control them. Instead, you may need to adjust your attitude from control to respect and your educational mode from instructing to advising.

A few tips for talking to your teen:

- Talk to her calmly and honestly about the dangers of not getting proper nutrition while she's still growing. Even if she acts angry, she will still hear you.
- Don't make a big deal about your teen's weight. If you do, it could cause him to eat out of rebellion or as a test to see if you still love him if he gains more weight.
- If your teenager is working on her weight and having a hard time with it, validate how difficult it is to change eating and exercise habits. Remind her that everyone enjoys food. Also, you might do a reality check to see if she's working too hard and

being too extreme in her efforts. If so, help her see that moderation is easier and more effective.
- Let your teenager have the last word.

Do's and Don'ts of Talking to Children of All Ages

Do	Don't
Provide information	Lecture
Make observations	Be judgmental
Ask questions	Have all the answers
Offer suggestions	Reprimand
Be honest	Be manipulative
Tread lightly	Nag
Provide support	Threaten
Praise their attributes	Criticize
Provide encouragement	Push

As with all parenting skills, learning to talk with your child about these delicate issues takes practice. Don't be afraid to try and don't be too hard on yourself if it doesn't work smoothly the first time. Keep practicing.

24

Nurturing Your Child's Self-Esteem

HELPING YOUR CHILD LOSE WEIGHT the healthy way means protecting her emotional, as well as physical, health. And when it comes to the emotional health of a child, self-esteem is at the core. Good self-esteem helps children feel comfortable about themselves and their bodies and gives them the confidence to try new things. Poor self-esteem can lead to depression or feelings of helplessness and failure.

As a parent, you do not bear full responsibility for your child's self-esteem, but what you say and do has a tremendous influence on how a child feels about herself. Unfortunately, many well-meaning parents inadvertently say things that can chip away at a child's self-esteem.

For example, nagging a child about what he eats or doesn't eat, belittling him for poor performance in a sport, or making comments about his weight in front of other people can be devastating to an overweight child's self-esteem.

What you say about other people's weight affects your youngster's view of himself, too. A child who hears you praise a thin person as having "a great body," while you refer to an overweight person as being "a fat slob," is likely to apply these standards to himself. Therefore, if your child feels overweight, he may deduce that you think he's a fat slob and come to think of himself in those terms as well.

It's also potentially damaging to have expectations for your offspring that they cannot attain. For example, if you set an unrealistic goal for a child's weight loss or allow her to choose one that she is unlikely to achieve, you're setting her up for failure. And when a child fails at something she's come to believe she can control, she will likely feel that the failure is her fault. Guilt, blame, and shame are all pathways to lowered self-esteem.

Depending upon how your youngster currently views herself, you'll want to either help her maintain her good self-image or try to help counteract her low self-esteem. First, praise your child's attributes and accomplishments. Congratulate her for good grades, tell her she's pretty, remind her that she has lots of good friends, point out her caring nature, or tell her how helpful she is around the house. Another way to maintain her self-esteem is to treat your overweight child the same as you treat your other children. For example, when you slice the birthday cake, don't give her a smaller piece than anyone else gets. You don't want her to feel inferior to her siblings just because she carries some extra weight.

Building healthy self-esteem doesn't involve hiding the truth from your child. Children can spot insincerity in an instant. Instead, be honest, but avoid negative or derogatory comments. For example, it's okay to acknowledge that your youngster is heavier than some other children. But at the same time, point out that everyone has different qualities. Some children are taller or shorter than others; some have red hair, while others have brown hair. Make it clear that these are differences that have nothing to do with a person's character. A child with blue eyes is no less valuable than one with brown eyes; and a child who's got more weight is no less lovable or worthwhile than one who is thinner.

What to Say if Your Child Is Being Teased

One of the most traumatic experiences for an overweight child is being teased by other children. If your child wants help dealing with classmates who are teasing him about his weight, you might offer him a two-step approach.

First, he should think of ways to answer back or tease the teaser about something. If the baiting persists, then he should simply ignore the comments. It's not necessarily better for your child to ignore the teasing from the very beginning. The risk with saying nothing when he's first teased is that the bully could interpret your child's silence as an indication that he's wounded him so deeply that he's paralyzed and can't do or say anything back. This would be a victory for the bully. However, snapping back initially and then, after a while, ignoring the bully to show that he has no power is more likely to make him stop teasing.

If the teasing at school is your child's first clue that he might be overweight, he may come home and say in a puzzled way, "Henry called me fatso." Depending upon your child's appearance, you may need to acknowledge that he has a little extra weight compared to other children. But it's also important to say, "It wasn't right for Henry to make fun of you. If it troubles you, I can help you. There are some things we can do to help you lose a little weight."

How to Talk to Family Members Who Make Insensitive Remarks

Criticism is extremely damaging to a child's self-esteem. And while family members may not mean to wound your child, their insensitive remarks are hurtful nonetheless.

The first step is to talk with family members and get their agreement not to discuss your child's weight, appearance, or eating habits. It is particularly important to have an understanding among members of your household that teasing and snide comments will not be tolerated. If they can't say something in support, they should refrain from saying anything at all.

However, it's a bit more difficult with relatives who are not part of your household. Grandparents, for example, may be worried about their granddaughter's being overweight and believe that by saying something to her, they can help influence her to lose weight. In this case, talk to your parent or parents about the issues of self-esteem we've discussed in this chapter. Also, reassure them that you're doing what is appropriate to help your child with her weight.

Unfortunately, you can't completely control the behaviors of others. So if the insensitive comments persist, you will have to turn your focus to your child and help her put the remarks into perspective. For example, you might say, "I know that Grandma told you that you won't find a boyfriend unless you're thin. That's the way Grandma remembers things from when she was young. I don't think it was the case then, and it's certainly not true now." You don't want your child to lose respect for your mother, but you do want to help her discount such negative comments.

Talking About Society's Views About Weight and Body Size

Seeing all of the thin bodies on television, in movies, and in magazines is a constant reminder to your chubby child that she's different. And because these media reflect many of the negative views our society holds about weight and body size, she soon gets the message that her shape is not desirable.

Although you can't shield your child from unrealistic body images or negative messages, you can help her to see them in a more realistic light. Some of the themes you may want to address in the course of television viewing include:

- *Striving for unrealistic body shapes and sizes is an exercise in futility.* You can tell your child that researchers say that only 1 in 10,000 females are biologically able to attain the model-thin bodies we see in the media.
- *Just because you may never look like a model or television star doesn't mean you can't attain a healthy weight and be physically fit.* This is a reality message that helps a child see that life is never "all or nothing." Her genetics may make it unlikely that she'll ever be a fashion model, but it doesn't mean that she can't be healthy and attractive.
- *You don't have to be thin to have the things you want in life.* This message can be tailored, as appropriate, to help your child see that you don't have to be thin to: (a) be attractive; (b) be a success in life; (c) have friends; (d) find a partner; (e) enjoy yourself; (f) all of the above.

What If Your Child Asks, "Am I Fat?"

You can start by responding to his question with the question, "What do you think?" And then, depending on whether he says "yes" or "no," you can follow with, "Why do you think that?" This way you'll have a somewhat better idea of your child's perceptions and feelings.

When you answer his question, your goal is threefold. First, be honest. For example, if your child is normal weight, say so. "I know you think you're fat, but you really aren't. No one thinks you're fat. You're a normal weight for your age and size and you look just fine."

If, on the other hand, he is somewhere between a little chubby and quite overweight, you can't deny it. Your child will know that you're not telling the truth. This is where the second goal comes in: Don't say your child is fat or use any other derogatory words. So instead of saying, "Yes, you're fat," it is probably more honest to say something like, "No, you're not fat, you just have a little extra weight. It's no big deal." Or if your child is really overweight, it's both truthful and kind to say, "No, I don't think you're fat, but you have put on some weight recently. If it bothers you, there are things we can do to help you lose some of the extra weight." You can even say, "Well, you are heavier than many children, and I've been thinking about it myself. Would you like me to help you try to lose some weight?"

The third goal is to assure your child that he is lovable and capable, regardless of his body shape or size. You may have to come right out and say it. For example, "I know that you're concerned about your weight, and I'm happy to help you try to control it. But I want you to know that I love you, and regardless of whether or not you lose weight, I'll still love you."

Going Shopping

Things you say to your child help nurture her self-esteem "from the inside out." There's also a way to improve your child's self-esteem "from the *outside* in" by helping your child look as attractive as possible. This is true for boys as well as girls, but it's especially important for preteen and teenage girls.

An effective way to enhance your child's appearance is to help her choose clothes that are flattering. First, don't get upset in the dressing room if she picks something that's not to your taste. Remember there is a generation gap between you. However, if you truly think an item is unbecoming, be truthful, but kind. One approach is to say that you think that particular style was designed for another type of body. You can even blame the designers by commenting,

"Why do they make these crazy clothes that only toothpicks can wear? This style doesn't look good on anyone."

Help your child buy clothes that make her look her best, in terms of both style and color. And help her see that although her body may not conform to society's notion of "perfection," she can still look good in clothes. If you see something on the rack that you think might suit her, you can always use the "try it, you might like it" approach, but don't push too hard. And when she tries on an outfit that really looks attractive on her, rave about it and mention that it's a good "style" for her.

It's no secret that growing up is stressful, and the stress of being overweight is an added burden for a child. Nurturing your youngster's self-esteem will help her feel happier and more confident while she's working on her weight.

25

When to Seek
Professional Help

REASONS FOR SEEKING PROFESSIONAL HELP can range from personal preference to absolute necessity. For example, you may know how to
swim, but decide to send your child to a swimming class instead of
trying to teach him yourself. In other circumstances, you may call a
professional because you lack the appropriate training to tackle the
job, such as tutoring your child in French when you took German in
school. But certain situations you encounter in your life won't go
away, and may get significantly worse if you don't seek professional
help. For example, you can't fill your own cavities or set your own
broken bones.

When it comes to helping your child lose weight the healthy way,
you may choose to seek professional guidance to make the task
easier or to be sure you're on the right track. On the other hand,
your child's problem or family circumstances may *require* you to get
help from a qualified professional. Whether the appropriate professional is a dietitian, fitness expert, psychologist, or other mental health
provider will depend upon your particular situation and your child's
individual needs.

Do You Need Help Implementing
Food-Related Strategies?

Concepts are easier to embrace than they are to put into action. Perhaps your efforts to help your child with her weight would be more
successful if you had a little help getting started. Or maybe you've

tried to make some changes and have run into roadblocks. In either case, consulting with a registered dietitian can make your job less frustrating and more effective. Whether it's one visit or several, a dietitian can help with a range of food-related issues, including:

- *Helping you properly assess the food behaviors of your child and your family.* If you filled out the food records and other assessments in part I, but had trouble analyzing them, a dietitian can be of service. He or she can help you accurately assess your child's eating behaviors and the family habits that may be contributing to his being overweight. Based on that information, the dietitian also can help you choose strategies that are most likely to work for you and your child.

- *Making sure that you're providing good nutrition for your child and family.* This may be particularly difficult if, for example, your child hates milk or won't eat vegetables. A dietitian can help you identify creative ways to ensure that your child gets good nutrition for proper growth.

- *Solving logistical problems.* Perhaps you're having trouble fitting low-fat eating into your life because your family eats out a lot or you have an unpredictable schedule. A problem-solving session could focus on developing strategies that will suit your lifestyle.

- *Helping you to be a better role model for your child.* If you have a personal history of yo-yo dieting, overeating, or poor nutrition, you may want to improve your own eating habits before embarking on a program to help your child. This is no easy task. So if you've had limited success in the past, you may want to get some help from a professional.

- *Adapting recipes to be lower in fat, sugar, and calories.* Whether you're a gourmet chef or a microwave wizard, you may need some assistance with making healthier dishes your family will enjoy. Here again, a dietitian can review your favorite recipes and suggest ways to cut fat and calories without sacrificing nutrition or taste.

For names of registered dietitians in your area who offer nutrition counseling, call the American Dietetic Association Nutrition Hotline at 1-800-366-1655 or go to www.eatright.org, their website, and click on "Find a Dietitian." Another alternative is to look in your local Yellow Pages under the heading "Dietitians" or "Nutritionists." Registered dietitians will have the initials R.D. after their names.

When it comes to titles, it's important to note that although registered dietitians who provide group or individual counseling often refer to themselves as "nutrition counselors" or "nutritionists," people with no training in nutrition can legally use these titles as well. Be sure that the nutrition counselor you choose is a registered dietitian or holds a master's degree (M.S.) or Ph.D. in dietetics or nutrition. Then confirm that he or she has experience in weight-loss counseling for children and families.

We suggest that you visit the dietitian first by yourself. Then you can discuss with him or her the merits of bringing your child to any subsequent sessions.

Does Your Child Want to Lose Weight, But Not With Your Help?

Sometimes, children, particularly teenagers, will take advice from anyone and everyone—except their parents. If your child wants to work on her weight, but fends off every attempt you make to help, maybe she'll listen to a professional. Offer to take your child to a registered dietitian, or if she's old enough, perhaps she can see the dietitian on her own.

Do You Need Help Incorporating Fitness Into Your Family's Life?

Adding exercise to the family agenda doesn't need to be complicated—everyone knows how to walk. However, if you want to introduce other kinds of activities that are new to you and your child, you may want to talk to an expert in fitness for children. Finding such a professional is not always easy. If your child's school has a physical education teacher, you could start there. Another possibility is to ask at your local YMCA or health club to see if any of their fitness trainers have experience with children.

From either source, you can get information about appropriate exercises and activity levels for your child, fitness programs in your community for children, and suggestions for motivating your child to be more active.

Are Family Dynamics Contributing to Your Child's Weight Problem?

Focus for a moment on the subtitle of this book, *A Family Approach to Weight Control*. Family support and praise are as important as low-fat foods to the success of your child's weight-loss efforts.

However, if you're not able to modify certain elements of the home environment that are contributing to your child's weight problem, it may be time to talk to a professional. For example, if you or your spouse are unable to stop nagging your child about his eating habits, or if family fights seem to trigger your youngster to eat more, counseling may help you identify the underlying problems and find ways to solve them.

Ask your child's pediatrician or your family physician for a referral to a mental health professional who does family therapy. You may be referred to a social worker (L.C.S.W.), a family counselor (M.F.T.), a psychologist (Ph.D.), or a psychiatrist (M.D.).

Did Your Child Start Gaining Weight After a Traumatic Experience?

If your child gained his extra weight rather suddenly, it may be that some traumatic experience triggered a change in his eating behavior. Think back to when he first started to gain weight. Does it correspond to a specific stressful event, such as the death of a family member, moving to a new town, or the arrival of his baby sister? Perhaps your youngster has been trying to cope with his emotional upset by eating.

You can start by talking with your child about the incident or experience you suspect might be bothering him. But when you discuss the situation with him, focus on the stressful event, not on his weight or eating. If you can get your child to talk about what's upsetting him, you may be able to help him resolve the conflict.

However, it's often difficult for a parent to uncover these kinds of issues or to help a youngster share painful feelings. That's where a therapist who works with children can be of assistance. A mental health professional knows how to help a child open up about what's troubling her. And if a traumatic experience is prompting your child to overeat, dealing with the emotional problem can help to resolve the eating problem as well.

Your doctor should be able to refer you to a mental health professional who specializes in children.

Is Your Child Extremely Overweight?

A youngster who is extremely overweight doesn't necessarily require professional help. All of the recommendations we've made in this book can help a child who is obese, as well as one who is just a little bit chubby. Although there's no denying that the more overweight your child is, the more work will be involved, we urge you not to give up too quickly. If, however, your child is quite overweight and hasn't responded to your efforts to help her lose weight or to the admonitions of her doctor, it may be time to seek professional help.

This is particularly true if your youngster's eating seems out of control—if he eats when he's not hungry and can't seem to stop. Or perhaps your child has a lot of stress in his life and he's eating excessively to try to relieve the tension. A professional may be able to uncover emotional causes of your child's eating.

If you suspect that an emotional problem may be contributing to your child being overweight, first try talking to a dietitian. If that doesn't help, the dietitian or your child's doctor can refer you to a mental health professional who works with children and families.

Not every extremely overweight child has psychological problems, but if your child does, it's important to seek help before an eating problem turns into an eating disorder.

Do You Think Your Child Might Have an Eating Disorder?

There's a fine line between an eating problem and an eating disorder, but there's also a world of difference. An eating problem is mostly about food, although it may involve some underlying psychological issues. An eating disorder, on the other hand, is a mental illness in which a severe distortion in eating behavior is the major observable symptom.

Eating disorders include anorexia nervosa, bulimia nervosa, and binge eating disorder. While these disorders all have different symptoms and somewhat varied warning signs, they share three common features: They indicate serious emotional problems; they pose serious risks to a child's physical and mental health; and they cannot be effectively treated or controlled without professional help. Adolescents are at particular risk for eating disorders, but children as young as eight years old may also be affected.

Anorexia nervosa is sometimes called the "starvation sickness" because people with this disorder starve themselves in order to become extremely thin. It is estimated that 1 in 500 adolescents suffers from anorexia. Anorexics severely restrict their food or resort to purging behaviors, such as induced vomiting or the misuse of laxatives, diuretics, or enemas, in order to lose and maintain an unnaturally low weight.

The health consequences of anorexia nervosa are varied and wide-ranging, including ulcers, heart problems, growth retardation, delayed puberty, and anemia. If anorexia is left untreated, it can result in death.

While most children who diet to lose weight do not become anorexic, restrictive dieting is the first step for those who do develop this eating disorder. With anorexia, dieting behavior becomes more and more compulsive as the individual struggles to exert control over her life by rigid control of her eating.

Usually, by the time an individual is diagnosed with anorexia nervosa, she is significantly underweight and intensely afraid of gaining weight or becoming fat. However, it may be possible to spot the early symptoms of anorexia before they result in excessive weight loss. If your child used to be more overweight but has recently been losing weight at a rapid pace, consider whether she also exhibits some of the warning signs listed on page 246—indicating that she may be in the beginning stages of anorexia.

More common among children, particularly adolescents, is bulimia nervosa, a disorder in which the individual has recurrent episodes of binge eating, followed by purging or other extreme behaviors, such as fasting or excessive exercising, to try to compensate for the bouts of overeating. Some estimates indicate that bulimia affects 1 to 3 percent of adolescents. They may binge and purge, most often by vomiting, once a day or several times a day. Many individuals with eating disorders alternate between anorexia and bulimia.

Low self-esteem is the hallmark of bulimia. Individuals with this condition are intensely embarrassed about their behavior, feeling great shame for both bingeing and purging.

A child with bulimia may be normal weight or somewhat overweight. However, if she purges by vomiting, she may appear chubby because of puffy "chipmunk" cheeks caused by enlargement of the salivary glands due to overstimulation. Other health conditions associated with bulimia nervosa include heart problems, abdominal pain, anemia, and erosion of the tooth enamel caused by the vomiting.

Binge eating disorder is a more recently documented eating disorder. Like bulimia, it involves recurring episodes of excessive eating, but they are not followed by purging or other behaviors to compensate for the binge. As a result, individuals with binge eating disorder may be average weight but most often are overweight.

Binge eating is distinguished from overeating in that the binges involve eating huge quantities of food, rapidly, and with a sense of losing control, until the individual becomes uncomfortably full. A binge eater often eats alone because of embarrassment and often feels depressed or guilty about bingeing.

If you suspect that your child has or may be developing an eating disorder, refer to the warning signs on page 246. A child with an eating disorder will not exhibit all of the warning signs, but most likely will display several of them. Early detection for eating disorders offers the best opportunity for treatment before more serious health problems occur.

This information is not meant to scare you or make you unduly concerned about your child. However, given the startling numbers of children, both girls and boys, who develop eating disorders, you cannot ignore the possibility that your child could have a more serious problem than being overweight.

If you suspect that your child may have one of the eating disorders we described, talk to your child's doctor right away. Do not wait until severe weight loss or a serious medical problem proves you right. An evaluation by a dietitian or mental health professional who is knowledgeable about eating disorders will likely be the first step in determining whether your child has an eating disorder. Treatment usually involves a combination of medical, psychological, and nutrition interventions for the child, as well as for appropriate members of the family.

Warning Sign	Anorexia Nervosa	Bulimia Nervosa	Binge Eating Disorder
Large, rapid weight loss	X	X	
Denies worry about low body weight	X		
Great fluctuations in body weight		X	X
Excessive or compulsive exercising	X	X	
Preoccupation with dieting and weight loss	X	X	X
Preoccupation with eating and food	X	X	X
Distorted body image; feels fat even when thin	X	X	
Wears big or baggy clothes or dresses in layers to hide body shape and/or weight loss	X	X	
Refuses to eat, eats tiny portions, and/or denies hunger	X	X	
Consumes unusually large quantities of food		X	X
Eats by herself or is secretive about food	X	X	X
Eats only a few types of foods	X	X	
Unusual food rituals, like chewing food and spitting it out	X	X	
Disappears after eating, usually to the bathroom		X	
Develops dental problems		X	
Has irregular menstrual cycles	X	X	
Has swollen salivary glands or puffy cheeks		X	
Complains of often feeling cold	X	X	
Is depressed, moody, or insecure	X	X	X
Purchases laxatives and/or diet pills	X	X	
Eliminates normal activities	X	X	X
Steals food or money to buy food		X	X

Needing professional help is not a sign of failure on your part or that of your child. Whether it's to learn how to make more nutritious low-fat meals, to help your child deal with stress, or for treatment of a serious eating disorder, seeking appropriate professional help is always a positive step.

26

Take One Step at a Time

THERE'S AN OLD AFRICAN PROVERB THAT SAYS, "No one tests the depth of a river with both feet." Making changes one step at a time and evaluating as you go along is a lot smarter than jumping in with both feet, only to find that the water's too deep or the current is too swift. Although making changes in your family's eating and exercise habits can seem as bumpy as white-water rafting, you can smooth out the ride if you make the changes moderate and just a few at a time.

Throughout the book, we've offered you hundreds of strategies, tips, and ideas for helping your child lose weight the healthy way. This last chapter is designed to help you identify the first steps you're going to take toward your goal. But before you can get started on your journey, you have to have a clear idea of where you're going.

Setting Goals

Establishing a long-range goal keeps you focused on your ultimate destination and helps you make choices along the way that support your objective. Here are three possible long-range goals to choose among—or you may have yet a different goal in mind.

Stop crash dieting. If your child is already trying to lose weight and is doing it by excessive dieting, your goal might be to help her work on her weight in a more healthy and effective way.

Prevent weight gain. As we've said all along, your youngster may not need to lose weight. It may be most appropriate to stabilize his weight, work on healthy eating habits, and let growth take care of the rest.

Begin to lose some weight. Depending upon your child's age, weight, and growth potential, losing some weight may be a realistic goal. But we urge you not to set a pound limit. Just start making changes and see how things go.

Starting With Baby Steps

Keep in mind that you won't need to follow *all* of our suggestions in order to help your child with her weight. We've given you a wide range of strategies on purpose, so you can choose the ones that are most appropriate for your child's needs and your family's lifestyle. But you will have to make *some* changes in food and activity patterns in order to help your child.

Fortunately, you can start with baby steps, changes that aren't particularly difficult for you and that your child won't even be aware of or care about. For example, she's not going to notice if you cut down on the amount of oil you use when stir-frying chicken or if you change from regular pancake syrup to a reduced-calorie version. And these changes do not require extra work on your part.

In time, you'll be able to take intermediate steps that involve greater change and that are likely to be noticed by your child. Perhaps serving sweets for dessert less often, or cooking just enough of a higher-fat entree so there's not enough for second helpings would be intermediate steps in your family. They might take some practice on your part, and you also may have to explain to your child that fruit is a dessert, too, and that "seconds" can be extra salad.

When it comes to giant-sized steps, don't even try. Some changes will be just too disruptive for your family. Besides, extreme changes aren't necessary to help your child lose weight the healthy way. Your child doesn't need to have a perfect diet or run marathons. She just has to take enough small steps to reach her goal.

Taking the First Step

It may be hard to rein in your enthusiasm now that you've got the knowledge to help your child. Or maybe you're overwhelmed with all of this new information and don't know where to start. Perhaps these thoughts will help:

- Don't try to do everything at once. Now that you have the knowledge, it's tempting to try to put it all into action right away. But taking one step at a time means making no more than a few changes at any one time.
- Success breeds success, so work on strategies you can accomplish comfortably. The first achievements may seem small, but they will form the foundation for future changes.
- Don't work on strategies that address problems you don't have. In other words, if your child doesn't eat ice cream very often, don't try to cut it down even more. Instead, work on reducing his twenty-five hours a week of television viewing.

The next sections focus on the three key areas for change: improving family eating behaviors, increasing family activity and exercise levels, and enhancing your parenting techniques. You may want to start by choosing one strategy in each of these areas or by concentrating in just one area.

Each area is broken down into several opportunities for change, and these are narrowed down to specific steps. Wherever applicable, we've also noted the chapter or chapters that offer more tips and ideas.

Improving Family Eating Behaviors

Improving eating behaviors is such a large area that we've separated it into five parts: at the supermarket, in the kitchen, scheduling for success, providing a more supportive environment for weight control, and eating away from home.

At the Supermarket

- Make a shopping list in advance and stick to it. *Refer to chapters 10 and 14 for more details.* Here are just a few steps to consider:

  Buy high-calorie treats only on the day they'll be eaten.
  Bring home smaller amounts of tempting high-calorie foods.
  Make sure there's enough variety in the foods you buy to prevent boredom.
- Read labels so you know what you're buying. *Refer to chapter 14 for a refresher on label reading.*

Find acceptable lower-fat products. *See chapter 13 for substitution ideas.*

Look for items with good nutrition.

Watch out for excessive sugar.

- Take your child shopping with you.

    Let your child pick some items, such as his favorite low-sugar cereal, yogurt, or fresh fruits and vegetables.

    Teach your youngster something new about good nutrition or label reading each time you go to the market.

- Buy convenience.

    Buy individual packages for easy, healthy snacks and bag lunches.

    Be careful that the convenience foods aren't higher in calories than you want.

In the Kitchen

- Prepare foods with less fat and sugar. *See chapter 15 for lots of tips.*

    Use less oil, margarine, and butter when cooking.

    Modify some of your existing recipes to be lower in fat and sugar. *See tips in chapter 13.*

    Try "mixing" as a way to reduce fat gradually. *Refer to chapter 15.*

    Increase frequency of fruits and vegetables. *There are lots of ideas in chapter 15.*

    To get even more creative ideas, buy a new low-fat cookbook or borrow one from the library. You also can try some of the recipes in the next section of this book.

- Serve smaller amounts of higher-calorie foods but don't cut them out completely.

    Try cooking just what your family needs for one meal.

    When you cook enough for two meals, put the second half away immediately in the refrigerator or freezer.

    Compensate for fewer high-fat foods by serving larger amounts of low-fat foods.

- Let your child help with meal planning and cooking if she's interested.

Let your child help you make the grocery list.
Choose age- and skill-appropriate tasks for her to contribute to
preparing and cooking food.

Scheduling for Success

- Schedule more regular meals. *See chapter 16 for specifics.*

  Don't let your child skip breakfast.
  Help your child make a nutritious lunch he likes so he won't buy
  junk food.
  You don't have to have dinner at the same time every day, just as
  long as your child knows when she can expect to eat.

- Plan healthy snacks. *Refer to chapters 10 and 16.*

  Include a mid-morning and a mid-afternoon snack as appropriate.
  Try including some protein in the snack if your child gets too
  hungry before the next meal.

- Eat more meals together.

  If you rarely eat dinner as a family, try to plan a family meal once
  or twice this week.
  Try having breakfast together on weekends.

- Work on "balancing acts." *Refer to chapter 11.*

  Try to balance food better on a daily basis.
  Focus on balancing high-fat favorites with acceptable lower-fat
  substitutes.
  Work on balancing empty calories with good nutrition.

Providing a More Supportive Environment for Weight Control

- De-fat the house. *Refer to chapters 10, 13, and 14.*

  Minimize the amount of high-fat and high-sugar foods that are in
  the house on a regular basis.
  Put tempting foods out of sight.
  Make nutritious foods easily available—wash the fruit and put it in
  a bowl on the table.
  If you want an extra sweet yourself, eat it during the day at work.

- Be a good role model. *See chapter 10 for more ideas.*

  Don't skip meals.
  Eat slowly, enjoying your food.
  Have fruit for dessert sometimes, instead of a sweet.

Eating Away From Home

- Work on restaurant strategies. *See chapter 17 for specifics.*

  If you eat out a lot, try going less often.
  When you eat out, try to be a good role model.
  Choose restaurants with plenty of healthy choices.

- Make more nutritious, lower-fat school lunches. *Refer to chapters 15 and 17.*

  Cut the fat in sandwiches.
  Find low-fat alternatives to chips and cookies.
  Boost the nutrition and minimize the empty sugar calories.

Increasing Family Activity and Exercise Levels

- Reduce sedentary habits. *Review chapter 18.*

  Negotiate to limit TV viewing and computer time.
  Use the car less often.

- Increase activities. *Look back at the ideas in chapter 19.*

  Shoot some baskets with your child after work.
  Use the stairs when alone and with your child.
  Take a Frisbee along on a family picnic.

- Increase exercise. *See chapters 19, 20, and 21.*

  Start taking a family walk after dinner.
  Rent or buy an aerobics tape especially for children.
  Let your child sign up for a team sport or an exercise class
    he'd enjoy.

Enhancing Your Parenting Techniques

- Adopt more positive attitudes. *See chapters 10, 22, 23, and 24 for more ideas.*

  Accept that change has to be gradual.
  Stay flexible—don't be a drill sergeant when it comes to food or exercise.
  Don't use food as a reward or punishment.
  Don't nag.

- Make mealtimes more pleasant. *Refer to chapter 10.*

  Don't try to control your child's every mouthful.
  Don't make your child clean her plate if she's had enough to eat.
  Don't express displeasure if your child doesn't eat a special dish you prepared.

- Nurture your child's self esteem. *See chapter 24.*

  If someone in your family is being insensitive to your overweight child, talk to that family member privately.
  The next time your child needs new clothes, use some of our tips about shopping.

Your First Steps

Now it's your turn. First, write down your long-range goal:

_____

Next, make note of the first steps you're going to take toward accomplishing that goal:

_____

_____

_____

_____

And after you've made those changes and they feel comfortable, write down the next steps you're going to make:

_____

_____

And the next steps:

_____

_____

_____

_____

Here's an example:

Goal: *To help Ellen stop gaining weight.*
First steps:

1. Buy more fresh fruit and fewer sweets the next time I go to the market.
2. Have a tasty, low-fat snack prepared and in the refrigerator for Ellen when she gets home from school.
3. Have dinner as a family on Friday night.
4. Ask Ellen if she wants to go with me when I walk the dog after work.

Put One Foot in Front of the Other

Sometimes progress is made by taking little baby steps, and other times it may be more like two steps forward and one step backward. No matter how slow the process seems, we encourage you to keep trying. Maybe these final thoughts will help you get started and keep going.

- *Any change in the right direction is progress.* Doing something is better than doing nothing.
- *Keep practicing—persistence pays off.* If you try something that doesn't work the first time, maybe it will work the second time, or the third time.

- *Reevaluate as you go along.* Maybe something doesn't work because it's not a good fit for you or your child. If so, try something else.
- *When the going gets rough, salvage something.* If your day falls apart and it's either pizza for dinner or nothing—at least don't order it with extra cheese and pepperoni.
- *There's no rush—you have plenty of time.* You're helping your child with her weight while she's young, which is a tremendous advantage. It means you've got lots of time to make changes and she's got lots of time to learn healthy lifestyle habits.
- *You can do it!*

PART VI

Recipes

IN DECIDING WHICH RECIPES to include in this book, we used three criteria: they had to be easy to prepare, they had to be low in fat and sugar, and they had to appeal to children. We gathered them from a variety of sources: Some are family favorites we have created over the years; others are adapted from cookbooks that we use regularly. We hope many of them will become family favorites in your house.

Breakfast/Brunch/Lunch

~~~~~~~

BREAKFAST SHAKE
Serves 1

Some children aren't hungry in the morning, but it's important for them to have something nourishing to start the day. A breakfast shake may be just the right solution.

$1/2$ cup skim milk
$1/2$ cup fruit (strawberries, bananas, etc.)
6 ounce low-fat yogurt (fruit flavor)
3 or 4 ice cubes
1 dash cinnamon and/or nutmeg

Place all ingredients except cinnamon or nutmeg in blender. Blend on high until creamy and smooth. Sprinkle with cinnamon and/or nutmeg.

Calories per serving: 239 calories
Percent calories from fat: 9%

〰〰〰〰

Breakfast Parfait
Serves 1

This fun, colorful breakfast parfait is easy to make. You can prepare it or let your child help with the layering.

½ cup low-fat granola
½ cup non-fat or low-fat vanilla or lemon yogurt
½ cup sliced strawberries or other fresh or canned fruit

Start with 1/4 cup granola in the bottom of a tall glass. Top with 1/4 cup yogurt and 1/4 cup fruit. Repeat the process for the second layer.

Calories per serving: 277 calories
Percent calories from fat: 13%

〰〰〰〰

Cinnamon-Raisin Scones
Serves 8, 1 scone per serving

These scones take just fifteen minutes to prepare and fifteen minutes to bake. They're great for a weekend treat. The only problem is that they are so delicious, it's hard to stop at one scone.

1¾ cups all-purpose flour
3 tablespoons sugar
1 tablespoon baking powder
2 teaspoons ground cinnamon
¼ teaspoon salt
¼ cup margarine, melted
¼ teaspoon orange peel
½ cup low-fat buttermilk
1 egg
2 teaspoons vanilla extract
⅓ cup raisins
3 tablespoons all-purpose flour
1 teaspoon sugar

Preheat the oven to 425° F. In a medium mixing bowl, combine the flour, sugar, baking powder, cinnamon, and salt. In another mixing bowl, combine the margarine, orange peel, low-fat buttermilk, egg, vanilla extract, and raisins. Add the buttermilk mixture to the flour mixture. Stir for 30 to 60 seconds, until the mixture gathers together into a ball. Sprinkle 3 tablespoons of flour onto a clean surface. With lightly dusted hands, knead the dough for 1½ to 2 minutes. Place kneaded dough on an ungreased baking sheet. Pat the dough out into an 8-inch circle. Sprinkle the circle with 1 teaspoon of sugar. With a pizza cutter, cut the circle into 8 triangular wedges. Separate the wedges from each other so they are not touching. Bake at 425° F for 15 minutes, until light golden brown.

Calories per serving: 209 calories
Percent calories from fat: 30%

Adapted from the *American Heart Association Kids' Cookbook.*

~~~~~~

CORNMEAL CHICKEN MUFFINWICHES
Serves 4, 2 muffins per serving

This "sandwich in a muffin" can be stored in an airtight plastic bag in the freezer for up to two months. Then pop a couple into a lunch bag in the morning and they will be thawed by noontime. If you want to serve them for dinner, they go great with a bowl of tomato soup.

> 8½ ounces packaged corn muffin mix
> 2 egg whites
> ⅓ cup skim milk
> 2 cups (8 ounces) coarsely chopped, cooked chicken, without skin
> 4 green onions, sliced
> ¼ teaspoon dried sage

Preheat the oven to 400° F. Prepare corn muffin mix according to package directions, but use egg whites for the egg and skim milk for the milk. Fold the chicken, green onions, and sage into the batter.

Spray 8 muffin cups with vegetable oil spray or line with paper bake cups. Spoon the batter into the cups. Bake 15 to 20 minutes or until a toothpick inserted near the center comes out clean. Cool. Serve warm or at room temperature.

Calories per serving (2 muffins): 307 calories
Percent calories from fat: 18%

Recipe from the *American Heart Association Quick and Easy Cookbook.*

Dinner

∿∿∿∿∿

Chunky Potato Soup
Serves 3, 1¼ cups per serving

This creamy potato soup is great on a wintry night. Serve with a salad and bread for a light but satisfying meal.

2 large baking potatoes (approximately 12 ounces each)
1 14½-ounce can chicken broth
2 tablespoons light sour cream
⅛ teaspoon ground black pepper
1 ounce reduced-fat cheddar cheese, grated
1 green onion, chopped
1 tablespoon imitation bacon bits

Bake the potatoes in an oven or microwave. Peel the potatoes. Cut one potato into 4 to 6 pieces. Put these in a blender with chicken broth and blend on high speed until smooth. Pour the potato mixture into a saucepan. Cut the second potato into ½ inch cubes. Stir diced potatoes, sour cream, and ground pepper into the saucepan. Cook the soup on low until hot and steaming. Do not boil. Ladle the soup into bowls and sprinkle with a choice of toppings (cheese, onion, bacon bits).

Calories per serving: 202 calories
Percent calories from fat: 13%

Recipe from the *American Heart Association Kids' Cookbook.*

~~~~~~

WANT MORE SALAD
Makes 4 servings

This salad is so crunchy and delicious, kids won't realize it's healthy. It's easy to put together and keeps well for two days in the refrigerator.

>   2 apples, cut in small chunks (Granny Smith or Macintosh are
>   particularly good)
>   3 stalks celery, chopped fine
>   1/4 cup raisins
>   7 ounces pineapple chunks in juice, drained well

Dressing

>   1/4 cup reduced-fat mayonnaise
>   1/4 cup plain nonfat yogurt
>   2 tablespoons orange juice
>   2 teaspoons sugar

Combine the first four ingredients in a salad bowl. Combine the dressing ingredients and pour over the fruit. Toss and refrigerate or serve.

Calories per serving: 170 calories
Percent calories from fat: 27%

Adapted from *All-American, Low-Fat Meals in Minutes,* by M.J. Smith.

〜〜〜〜

CHICKEN ENCHILADAS
Serves 4, 2 enchiladas per serving

An easy make-ahead meal—even easier if you've got leftover chicken breast. While the casserole is in the oven, make a green salad or fruit salad to accompany it.

½ pound boneless chicken breast, cooked, skinned, and shredded (approximately 1 whole breast)
1 medium onion, chopped (½ cup)
1 small can creamed corn (9 ounces)
4 ounces reduced-calorie cheddar cheese, shredded (about 1 cup)
1 10-ounce can enchilada sauce
½ cup water
8 6-inch corn tortillas

Preheat the oven to 350° F. In a medium bowl, combine the chicken, onion, corn, and half of the shredded cheese. Set the mixture aside.

In a skillet, combine the enchilada sauce and water, and heat the sauce to boiling. Place a tortilla into the sauce. When the tortilla is limp, remove it from the skillet, letting the excess sauce drain back into the pan. Place the tortilla on a platter and spoon a generous ¼ cup of chicken-corn-cheese filling across its diameter. Roll up the tortilla, and set it seam side down in a 9 × 13-inch baking pan or shallow casserole. Repeat this procedure with the remaining tortillas, arranging them in the pan in a single layer. Pour the remaining sauce over the rolled tortillas, sprinkle the remaining cheese over them, cover the pan or casserole with foil, and bake at 350° F for 15 minutes. Remove the foil and bake the enchiladas for another 5 minutes, or until they are heated through and lightly browned.

Calories per serving: 365 calories
Percent calories from fat: 20%

Adapted from *Jane Brody's Good Food Book.*

~~~~~~

PINEAPPLE CHICKEN
Serves 4

An easy, one-pot entree. While the chicken is cooking, you can make some rice or noodles to go with it.

1 10-ounce can pineapple chunks, in juice
1 cup chopped onions
¼ cup chopped tomatoes
2 tablespoons brown sugar
2 tablespoons apple cider vinegar
2 garlic cloves, minced
½ teaspoon cinnamon
¼ teaspoon cloves
¼ teaspoon ground pepper
1 pound boneless, skinless chicken breast, cut into 2-inch chunks
2 teaspoons cornstarch
1 tablespoon water

Combine first 9 ingredients in a Dutch oven or heavy pot. Bring to a boil, uncovered, and cook, stirring occasionally, for 10 minutes. Stir in the chicken and return the mixture to a boil. Reduce heat and cover the pot. Simmer for 15 minutes. Mix cornstarch and cold water and add to the pot. Cook, over medium heat, until sauce bubbles and thickens. Serve over rice or noodles.

Calories per serving: 295 calories
Percent calories from fat: 12%

~~~~~~

SAVORY CHICKEN-VEGETABLE STEW
Serves 3

This hearty recipe is somewhat like a thick soup, but because it's so satisfying, we're calling it a stew. Serve with a green salad and French bread, for a great winter's meal. The recipe can be doubled.

½ cup chopped onion
½ cup chopped carrots
½ cup chopped celery
⅔ cup sliced mushrooms
1 can corn, drained (8–10 ounces)
16 ounces chicken broth (1 pint)
3 ounces dried bow-tie pasta
1 teaspoon dried tarragon
½ pound boned chicken breasts, skinned and cut into 1-inch
    cubes
1¼ cups 1% milk
2 teaspoons cornstarch

In a Dutch oven or heavy saucepan, boil the onion, carrots, celery, mushrooms, and ¼ cup of the broth. Stir occasionally and cook until the liquid evaporates and the vegetables brown a bit. Add the remaining broth and bring to a boil. Stir in the pasta and tarragon. Bring to a boil again, over medium-high heat, and continue to cook, covered, until the pasta is barely tender, about 8 minutes. Stir in the chicken. Add cornstarch to the milk, mix well, and add to the pot. Bring to a simmer, stirring occasionally, and cook for about 6 more minutes, until the stew has thickened. Season to taste with salt and pepper.

Calories per serving: 355 calories
Percent calories from fat: 17%

~~~~~~

MUSTARD CHICKEN
Serves 4

It doesn't get any easier than this. And the mustardy topping adds just the right amount of zip to the juicy chicken breasts.

4 skinless, boneless chicken breast halves
4 teaspoons Dijon mustard, or other mustard
4 teaspoons reduced-calorie mayonnaise
Pepper to taste

Preheat the broiler to high. Place breast halves between two sheets of wax paper and pound lightly with a mallet to flatten slightly. Spray a baking dish, large enough to hold the chicken breasts comfortably, with vegetable oil spray. Sprinkle each breast with pepper and arrange, skinned side up, on the baking dish. Do not overlap. Blend the mustard and mayonnaise. Spread equally over the breast halves. Broil chicken, 12 inches from the source of heat, for about 15 minutes, until the tops are brown and the chicken is cooked through. If you can't lower your broiler pan so that the chicken is at least 12 inches from the heat, lower the pan as far as you can and cook the chicken at 375° F.

Calories per serving: 164 calories
Percent calories from fat: 29%

Adapted from *Craig Claiborne's Gourmet Diet.*

∿∿∿∿∿

SWEET-AND-SOUR CHICKEN WITH VEGETABLES
Serves 2 to 3

Although it looks like a lot of ingredients, this recipe goes together quickly. It's got a great Oriental flavor—perfect over rice.

    12 ounces chicken breasts, boned and skinned
    4 teaspoons reduced-sodium soy sauce
    1 teaspoon sesame oil
    1-inch piece of fresh ginger
    ½ teaspoon minced garlic
    2 tablespoons brown sugar
    2 tablespoons dry sherry
    2 tablespoons cider vinegar
    2 tablespoons ketchup
    3 tablespoons water
    2 red onions, sliced thin (approximately 3 cups)
    16 ounces canned chopped tomatoes, drained
    1 tablespoon cornstarch

Wash and dry the chicken breasts and place them in a pan lined with aluminum foil. Mix together 1 teaspoon soy sauce and the sesame oil and brush on both sides of the chicken. Broil as close to the heat source as possible, about 10 minutes, turning once. Meanwhile, coarsely grate the ginger and mix it together with the garlic, the remaining 3 teaspoons of soy sauce, brown sugar, sherry, vinegar, ketchup, and 2 tablespoons water in a pot large enough to hold the chicken and vegetables. Bring the sauce to a boil. Stir in the onion and cook over medium heat. Add tomatoes and cook for 3 to 5 minutes. While the mixture cooks, cut cooked chicken into small chunks, and mix cornstarch with 1 tablespoon of water to form a smooth paste. When the onions are tender, stir in the cornstarch mixture and cook until the sauce thickens slightly. Stir in cooked chicken and heat through. Serve over rice.

Calories per serving: 360 calories
Percent calories from fat: 14%

Adapted from *20 Minute Menus* by Marian Burros.

~~~~~~~

Sweet and Sour Turkey Meatloaf
Serves 4

Be sure to buy ground turkey *breast* for this recipe, not just ground turkey. The difference in fat is substantial because ground turkey includes the turkey skin. The recipe can be doubled.

> 1 pound ground turkey breast
> 1 small onion, finely chopped
> 1/3 cup fine dry bread crumbs
> 1 egg, beaten
> 1 1/2 teaspoons dried parsley
> 1/4 cup ketchup
> 1/8 teaspoon ground pepper

Topping

> 1/4 cup apricot preserves
> 1 tablespoon brown sugar
> 1 tablespoon Dijon-style mustard

Mix the first 7 ingredients together well. Form a firm 6-inch round loaf and place it in the middle of a 10-inch round platter or pie plate. Cover with the topping. Microwave on high for approximately 14 minutes, rotating after 7 minutes. Meatloaf will be done when a thermometer inserted in the center registers 145° to 155° F. Let it stand for 5 minutes before slicing.

Calories per serving: 285 calories
Percent calories from fat: 9%

~~~~~~

Pasta Pie
Serves 4

This "pie" uses low-fat, fresh angel-hair pasta (from the refrigerated section) to form its crust. It is quick and easy to prepare, and while it bakes, you can make a salad to go along with it.

1/4 cup water
1 egg white
4 ounces fresh angel-hair (capellini) pasta (uncooked)
1/3 cup grated Parmesan cheese
8 ounces leanest ground beef
1/2 cup chopped onion
3/4 cup low-fat, meatless spaghetti sauce
3/4 cup shredded part-skim mozzarella cheese

Preheat the oven to 350° F. Lightly spray a 9-inch pie plate with vegetable oil spray. In a medium bowl, combine the water and egg white. Stir until well combined. Stir in uncooked pasta and Parmesan cheese. Place the pasta mixture in the pie plate. Press the mixture against the bottom and slightly up the sides of the pie plate to form an even crust. Set aside.

In a large skillet, cook ground beef and onion over medium-high heat until the meat is brown and the onion is tender, about 5 minutes. Place the cooked meat mixture in a colander and rinse it under hot water. Drain well. Wipe the skillet with a paper towel to remove fat. Return the meat mixture to the skillet. Stir in the spaghetti sauce; heat through, about 3 minutes. Spoon the meat mixture over the pasta crust. Bake, uncovered, for 20 minutes. Sprinkle with mozzarella cheese and bake about 5 minutes more or until cheese melts. Let stand 5 minutes, then cut into 4 wedges and serve.

Calories per serving: 270 calories
Percent calories from fat: 35%

Adapted from the *American Heart Association Quick and Easy Cookbook.*

~~~~~~

TACO CASSEROLE
Serves 6

This dish always gets rave reviews—no one even notices that it has beans in it.

    1 15-ounce can kidney beans, processed smooth in blender
    1 pound leanest ground beef, browned and drained
    1/2 teaspoon garlic powder
    1/2 teaspoon cumin
    1/4 teaspoon cayenne (optional)
    8 ounces tomato sauce
    1/4 cup chopped onion
    4 to 6 corn tortillas, cut into triangles
    2 ounces reduced-fat cheddar cheese, grated
    Dash chili powder for garnish (optional)

Preheat the oven to 375° F. Spray a 9 × 13-inch dish or two 8 × 8-inch baking dishes with nonstick cooking spray. Spread processed beans onto bottom of the prepared pan. Combine the browned meat with the garlic, cumin, cayenne, and tomato sauce. Spread over beans. Top with the onion, tortilla triangles, and cheese. Sprinkle chili powder on top. Bake for 30 minutes. Remove from oven and let stand 5 minutes. Serve with chopped lettuce and tomato. This may be assembled and frozen for later baking.

Calories per serving: 300 calories
Percent calories from fat: 20%

Adapted from *All-American, Low-Fat Meals in Minutes,* by M.J. Smith.

~~~~~~~

SWEET AND SOUR BARBECUED STEAK
Serves 6

This recipe will satisfy the meat-lovers in your house, but without the fat content of most steaks. London broil is one of the leanest steaks you can choose. The recipe calls for barbecuing, but you also can broil the steak (if it's fairly thin) or bake it (if it's thicker).

> 1/3 cup cider vinegar
> 1/4 cup honey
> 1/4 cup reduced-sodium soy sauce
> 1 clove garlic, minced or pressed
> 1/8 teaspoon liquid hot pepper seasoning
> 1 London broil (about 1 1/2 pounds)

In a small pan, combine vinegar, honey, soy sauce, garlic, and hot pepper seasoning. Place over medium heat and cook, stirring often, until the honey is dissolved and the mixture is well blended (about 5 minutes). Let cool slightly. Trim and discard any fat from the meat; place the steak in a shallow bowl or baking dish. Pour the vinegar mixture over the steak, cover, and refrigerate for at least 4 hours, or until the next day, turning the steak once or twice.

Remove the steak from the marinade and drain briefly, reserving the marinade. Spray a barbecue grill with cooking spray. Place the steak on the grill 4 to 6 inches above a solid bed of medium coals. Grill, turning once and basting often with some of the marinade, until done to your liking when slashed. While the steak is cooking, in a small pan, boil the remaining marinade over high heat until reduced to about 1/2 cup. Transfer the steak to a carving board and cut it across the grain into thin, slanting slices. Accompany with marinade.

Calories per serving: 265 calories
Percent calories from fat: 23%

Recipe from *Sunset Light Cuisine.*

~~~~~

BEEF AND VEGETABLE STIR-FRY
Serves 6

This delicious, low-fat stir-fry dish is made with the leanest beef (top round) and using no added oil or butter. It has a delicate sweet and sour flavor. The recipe calls for onions, carrots, and mushrooms, but you can use or add whatever fresh vegetables your family likes.

1/3 cup brown sugar, firmly packed
2 tablespoons cornstarch
1/4 cup cider vinegar
4 tablespoons reduced-sodium soy sauce
1 1/2 pounds top round steak
1 large onion, thinly sliced
1 1/2 cups thinly sliced carrots
1 1/2 cups thinly sliced mushrooms
1 cup water

In a small bowl, combine the brown sugar, cornstarch, vinegar, and soy sauce. Set aside. Trim and discard all visible fat from the meat. Cut it into thin, slanting slices (1/8 to 1/4 inch thick). In a large, nonstick frying pan or wok, cook the meat strips, a few at a time, stirring until well browned. Lift out the meat as it browns and set aside. When all of the meat is cooked, add the onion and carrots and 1/2 cup of water to pan. Stir well, cover, and cook, stirring occasionally, for approximately 8 minutes, until carrots are just tender crisp. Add the mushrooms and remaining 1/2 cup of water, and cook one more minute. Stir the cornstarch mixture and add it to the vegetables along with the meat. Cook, stirring, until the sauce boils and thickens. Serve immediately over rice.

Calories per serving: 310 calories
Percent calories from fat: 20%

~~~~~~~

TUNA NOODLE CASSEROLE
Serves 4

This is a low-fat version of an old-fashioned favorite.

1 can Healthy Request Cream of Mushroom Soup (10³/₄ ounces)
6 ounces chunk white, water-packed tuna, drained
1 teaspoon Worcestershire sauce
8 ounces wide noodles, cooked until just tender
¹/₂ ounce potato chips, crushed

Preheat the oven to 350° F. Mix the first 3 ingredients together in a 1¹/₂-quart casserole that has been sprayed with nonstick cooking spray. Add the noodles and mix thoroughly. Top with crushed potato chips and bake for approximately 30 minutes, or until brown and bubbly.

Calories per serving: 324 calories
Percent calories from fat: 12%

~~~~~~~

GOLDEN BAKED FISH
Serves 6

This crispy fish recipe can be made with filet of sole, rockfish, or other fish filets. Serve it with the yogurt-dill sauce on the side.

1 egg
1 tablespoon nonfat milk
¹/₂ cup fine dry bread crumbs (plain or seasoned)
4 tablespoons grated Parmesan cheese
1¹/₂ pounds filet of sole or other fish filets (¹/₄- to ¹/₂-inch thick)

Line a shallow 9 × 12-inch baking pan with foil and spray with vegetable spray. Place the empty pan in the oven and preheat to 500° F. Meanwhile, beat the egg and milk in a shallow pan until blended; mix bread crumbs and cheese in another shallow pan or on wax paper. Cut the fish into serving-size pieces, if necessary. Dip the fish first into the egg mixture, then into the crumb mixture, coating well on all sides. When the pan is hot, arrange the fish on it in a single layer. Bake, uncovered, until the fish is opaque in the center when tested with a knife (7 to 10 minutes). Serve with yogurt sauce.

Yogurt Sauce

   1 cup plain yogurt
   1/2 teaspoon dill weed
   1/2 teaspoon Dijon mustard
   1/3 cup chopped green bell pepper, cucumber, or dill pickle
   1/2 cup thinly sliced green onions (including tops)

Combine the ingredients in a medium-size bowl; stir until well combined. Set aside. If made ahead, cover and refrigerate for a day or two.

Calories per serving: 150 calories
Percent calories from fat: 19%

Adapted from *Sunset Light Cuisine.*

〜〜〜〜〜

TERIYAKI FISH KABOBS
Serves 3 to 4

Fish is more fun for kids when it's on skewers. The cook will like this recipe because it cooks quickly in the microwave. Serve with rice for an easy, delicious meal.

   1/4 cup reduced-sodium soy sauce
   1 tablespoon lemon juice
   1 teaspoon sesame oil
   2 cloves of garlic, minced
   4 teaspoons grated fresh ginger
   1 pound firm, fresh fish—halibut, swordfish, or tuna
   1 can pineapple chunks (8 ounces)
   16 fresh mushrooms, small (or 8 medium, cut in half)
   1/2 red bell pepper

In a medium-size bowl, combine the first 5 ingredients. Cut fish into 16 cubes (about 1-inch square) and add to the marinade, stirring to coat. Cover and refrigerate for 30 minutes. Meanwhile, prepare the fruits and vegetables: drain the pineapple, wash and trim the mushrooms, and cut the bell pepper into 16 squares. Thread the fish, pineapple, mushrooms, and pepper onto 8 bamboo skewers—two of each per kabob. Place the kabobs in a 9 × 13-inch microwave-safe baking dish. Pour the marinade evenly over the kabobs. Cover with wax paper and microwave on high for 3 minutes; turn kabobs over and microwave another 3 to 5 minutes or until fish is done.

Calories per serving: 330 calories
Percent calories from fat: 17%

~~~~~~

PANTRY CASSEROLE
Serves 6

This is an easy-to-put-together casserole. Chances are the ingredients are already in your cupboard and refrigerator. Also, it can be prepared a day or two in advance of baking.

3 cups cooked brown or white rice (1 cup raw)
2 cups corn kernels (approximately 10 ounces)
1 small onion, finely chopped (1/2 cup)
6 ounces reduced-fat sharp cheddar cheese, grated
1 1/2 cups nonfat or 1% milk
1 teaspoon chili powder, or more, to taste
1/4 teaspoon cumin
1/4 teaspoon freshly ground black pepper
Sprinkle paprika

In a large mixing bowl, combine all the ingredients except the paprika and mix them well. Pour the ingredients into a 2-quart casserole that has been sprayed with nonstick cooking spray. Sprinkle with paprika, and bake the casserole in a 350° F oven for 45 minutes.

Calories per serving: 260 calories
Percent calories from fat: 22%

Adapted from *Jane Brody's Good Food Book.*

~~~~~~~

LIGHT & EASY MACARONI & CHEESE
Serves 3

Kids love macaroni and cheese, so here's a way to serve their favorite with less fat. And don't worry, they won't miss it a bit.

1 package Macaroni & Cheese Dinner (7.25 ounces)
¼ cup 1% milk

Cook the macaroni as directed on the package. Drain well. Return to the pan. Add milk and Cheese Sauce Mix from the package. Mix well. Makes about 3 cups.

Calories per serving: 290 calories
Percent calories from fat: 9%

Vegetables

~~~~~~~

DRESSED-UP GREEN BEANS
Serves 4

Dressing up vegetables is one way to make them more appealing to children. Try these green beans on your children—they might just like them.

1 9-ounce package frozen green beans (or fresh)
1 cup diced tomato (about 1 large, or 2 small)
½ cup diced celery
2 garlic cloves, minced or pressed
½ teaspoon dried oregano leaves

Combine all ingredients in a saucepan and bring to a boil, separating beans with a fork as they thaw. Reduce heat, cover, and simmer about 5 minutes, or until beans are tender, but still crisp.

Calories per serving: 30
Percent calories from fat: zero

~~~~~~

HONEY CARROTS
Serves 4

This recipe is a real kid-pleaser. The brown sugar and honey add just enough sweetness to the carrots for children, but not too much for adult taste buds.

    8 ounces baby carrots, prewashed
    1 teaspoon margarine
    1 tablespoon brown sugar
    1 tablespoon honey
    2 tablespoons finely chopped parsley (optional)

Steam the carrots until just tender. Pour off liquid. Return the carrots to the pot with margarine, brown sugar, and honey. Cook over low heat, turning the carrots frequently until well glazed. Sprinkle with parsley, if desired, and serve immediately.

Calories per serving: 65 calories
Percent calories from fat: 14%

Adapted from the *American Heart Association Cookbook.*

~~~~~~

OVEN FRENCH "FRIES"
Serves 6

A great way to serve French "fries" without all the fat. These do take up to an hour to get crispy, so put them in the oven first and then fix the rest of the meal.

    6 medium potatoes, peeled
    1 tablespoon vegetable oil
    1 teaspoon garlic powder
    ¼ teaspoon salt

Slice the potatoes lengthwise. Make them as thick or as thin as you like (thinner will be crispier). Combine the oil, garlic, and salt in a large bowl. Add the potatoes and toss with your hands to coat.

Place on two cookie sheets, sprayed with nonstick cooking spray. Bake at 400° F for 45 to 60 minutes, turning several times, until well browned.

Calories per serving: 190 calories
Percent calories from fat: 9%

~~~~~~

CREAMY MASHED SWEET POTATOES
Serves 4

This easy recipe makes a great side dish for chicken or turkey. Why not add it to your Thanksgiving menu?

1 1/2 pounds sweet potatoes, peeled and cut into 2-inch pieces
1/2 cup nonfat yogurt
1/2 teaspoon grated nutmeg
1/4 teaspoon freshly ground black pepper
1/4 teaspoon salt
1 tablespoon brown sugar
1 teaspoon lemon juice

Place the sweet potatoes in a 2-quart, microwave-safe casserole with a 1/2 cup of water. Cover tightly with a lid or plastic wrap turned back slightly. Microwave on "high" for 10 to 12 minutes (or more), until tender, stirring once. With a potato masher, electric beaters, or food processor, mash the sweet potatoes with their cooking water until they are smooth. Stir in the remaining ingredients.

Calories per serving: 270 calories
Percent calories from fat: 3%

Recipe from *Home Cooking in Minutes* by Thelma Snyder and Marcia Cone-Esaki.

Desserts

∿∿∿∿∿

PINK APPLESAUCE
Serves 5, 1/2 cup per serving

This is a fun, fat-free dessert. The pink color comes from cinnamon "red-hot" candies. Look for them in the cake decorating section at the supermarket.

    1 24-ounce jar unsweetened applesauce
    2 tablespoons cinnamon "red-hot" candies
    ¼ teaspoon ground cinnamon

Combine applesauce, candies, and cinnamon in a medium saucepan. Stir the mixture with a wooden spoon over medium heat for 3 to 4 minutes, or until candies are melted. Serve warm or cover and refrigerate to serve chilled.

Calories per serving: 70 calories
Percent calories from fat: zero

Adapted from the *American Heart Association Kids' Cookbook.*

∿∿∿∿∿

FROZEN YOGURT POPS
Makes 8 pops

Children can help prepare these easy-to-make yogurt pops. They'll also like helping decide what combination of fruit juice and yogurt to try.

    1 6-ounce can frozen orange, grape, or apple juice concentrate
    ¾ cup water
    1 cup vanilla- or fruit-flavored low-fat yogurt

In a blender or food processor, whirl the juice concentrate, water, and yogurt until well blended. Divide the mixture evenly among eight 3-ounce paper drinking cups. Cover the cups and set in the freezer until partially frozen (about 1½ hours), then insert a wooden stick in each cup. Freeze until firm (about 2 hours).

Calories per serving: 70 calories
Percent calories from fat: 5%

Recipe from *Sunset Light Desserts.*

∿∿∿∿∿

MICROWAVE "BAKED" APPLES
Serves 4

These baked apples can be a delicious, no-fat dessert or part of a weekend breakfast.

    4 medium-size tart baking apples (Granny Smith, Rome)
    4 tablespoons raisins
    4 tablespoons brown sugar
    4 teaspoons orange juice
    4 teaspoons lemon juice
    4 teaspoons granulated, white sugar
    1 teaspoon ground cinnamon

Remove the apple cores to within ½ inch of the bottoms. Peel a 1-inch strip around the top of each apple and pierce the sides 4 times each with a fork (to allow steam to escape). Place each apple in a microwave-safe custard cup or around the edge of a 9-inch round microwave-safe cooking dish. Spoon 1 tablespoon of the raisins, 1 tablespoon of the brown sugar, and 1 teaspoon of the orange juice into the cavity of each apple. Sprinkle each with lemon juice, sugar, and cinnamon. Cover with plastic wrap turned back slightly. Microwave on high for 3 minutes, rotate dish(es), and microwave for an additional 3 minutes. If not soft enough, cook for 1 more minute. Spoon juices over apples. If serving warm, allow the apples to cool for 10 to 15 minutes. Or chill and serve cold.

Calories per serving: 180 calories
Percent calories from fat: 2%

Adapted from *Home Cooking in Minutes* by Thelma Snyder and Marcia Cone-Esaki.

~~~~~~

CHOCOLATE CRISPY TREATS
Makes 32 squares

This adaptation of a traditional kid-pleaser is easy to make and low in fat.

1/4 cup corn syrup
1 tablespoon margarine or low-fat margarine
1 bag marshmallows (10 1/2 ounces)
3 cups toasted rice cereal
3 cups toasted chocolate rice cereal

Spray a 13 × 9 × 2-inch baking pan with vegetable oil. Set aside. In a large saucepan or Dutch oven, cook the corn syrup and margarine over medium-low heat until the margarine melts, about 3 minutes. Add marshmallows and stir until completely melted, about 5 minutes. Remove from heat.

Add cereals and stir until well coated. Transfer to the baking pan. Spray the back of a metal spoon with vegetable oil. Use it to press mixture evenly into the prepared pan. Cover and refrigerate at least 30 minutes. Cut into 32 bars. Bars can be stored, covered tightly in the refrigerator, for up to 1 week.

Calories per serving: 60 calories
Percent calories from fat: 8%

From the *American Heart Association Quick and Easy Cookbook.*

~~~~~~

FROZEN YOGURT BANANA POPS
Makes 6

Kids can help with the preparation of this fun snack. It is a two-step process, so allow enough time.

  3 bananas, firm, green tipped
  1 cup flavored low-fat yogurt
  1 cup toasted rice or other cereal (crushed into small pieces if
    needed)

Peel bananas and cut in half crosswise. Insert a flat wooden stick into the cut end of each half. Dip the banana halves in yogurt to coat completely. Place the banana halves slightly apart on a baking sheet lined with wax paper. Cover with plastic wrap and freeze until the coating is firm (about 1 hour). Meanwhile, spread cereal on a baking sheet. Dip each banana in the yogurt again, then roll in the cereal. Return to the baking sheet, cover, and freeze until the coating is firm. Before serving, let stand at room temperature for about 5 minutes.

Calories per serving: 100 calories
Percent calories from fat: 4%

References and Supporting Research

Part I. First Assess Your Child

American Academy of Pediatrics, Committee on Nutrition. *Pediatric Nutrition Handbook, 4th Edition*, American Academy of Pediatrics, Elk Grove Village, IL. 1998

Barnes, HV. "Physical growth and development during puberty." *Medical Clinics of North America.* November 1975

Bouchard, C, et al. "The response to long-term overfeeding in identical twins." *The New England Journal of Medicine.* May 1990

Dietz, WH, and Bellizzi, MC. "Introduction: the use of body mass index to assess obesity in children." *American Journal of Clinical Nutrition.* July 1999

Faith, MS, et al. "Evidence for independent genetic influences on fat mass and body mass index in a pediatric twin sample." *Pediatrics.* July 1999

Feunekes, G, et al. "Food choice and fat intake of adolescents and adults: associations of intakes within social networks." *Preventive Medicine.* September–October 1998

Gillespie, A, and Achterberg, C. "Comparison of family interaction patterns related to food and nutrition." *Journal of the American Dietetic Association.* April 1989

Guo, S, and Chumlea, W. "Tracking of body mass index in children in relation to overweight in adulthood." *American Journal of Clinical Nutrition.* July 1999

Guo, S, et al. "The Predictive value of childhood body mass index values for overweight at age 35y." *American Journal of Clinical Nutrition.* April 1994

Gustafson-Larson, A, and Terry, R. Weight-related behaviors and concerns of fourth-grade children. *Journal of the American Dietetic Association.* July 1992

Hood, MY, et al. "Parental eating attitudes and the development of obesity in children. The Framingham Children's Study." *International Journal of Obesity Related Metabolic Disorders.* October 2000

Khamis, HJ. "Predicting adult stature without using skeletal age." *Pediatrics.* October 1994

Kuehneman, T, et al. "Comparability of four methods for estimating portion sizes during a food frequency interview with caregivers of young children." *Journal of the American Dietetic Association.* May 1994

Lake, JK, et al. "Child to adult body mass index in the 1958 British birth cohort: associations with parental obesity." *Archives of Disease in Childhood.* November 1997

Maffeis, C, et al. "Influence of diet, physical activity and parents' obesity on children's adiposity: a four-year longitudinal study." *International Journal of Obesity Related Metabolic Disorders.* August 1998

Nader, P. "The Role of the Family in Obesity Prevention and Treatment." *Prevention and Treatment of Childhood Obesity.* The New York Academy of Sciences, New York. 1993

Quek, CM, et al. "Parental body mass index: a predictor of childhood obesity?" *Annals of Academic Medicine Singapore.* May 1993

Strauss, RS, and Knight, J. "Influence of the home environment on the development of obesity in children." *Pediatrics.* June 1999

Stucky-Ropp, R, and DiLorenzo, T. "Determinants of exercise in children." *Preventive Medicine.* November 1993

Stunkard, A, et al. "The body-mass index of twins who have been reared apart." *New England Journal of Medicine.* May 1990

U.S. Department of Health and Human Services, Centers for Disease Control. "CDC Growth Charts: United States." June 2000

USDA Center for Nutrition Policy and Promotion. "Profile of Overweight Children." May 1999

Whitaker, RC, et al. "Predicting obesity in young adulthood from childhood and parental obesity." *New England Journal of Medicine.* September 1997

Part II. Children Are Different

Barlow, SF, and Dietz, WH. "Obesity evaluation and treatment: expert committee recommendations." *Pediatrics.* September 1998

Eptstein, L, et al. "Effect of weight loss by obese children on long-term growth." *American Journal of Diseases of Children*. October 1993

Epstein, L, et al. "Treatment of pediatric obesity." *Pediatrics*. March 1998

Hardy, SC. "Fat and cholesterol in the diet of infants and young children: implications for growth, development, and long-term health." *Journal of Pediatrics*. November 1994

Mallick, MJ. "Health hazards of obesity and weight control in children: a review of the literature." *American Journal of Public Health*. January 1993

Pugliese, M. "Fear of obesity: A cause of short stature and delayed puberty." *New England Journal of Medicine*. September 1983

Part III. Focus on Food

American Dietetic Association. "Dietary guidance for healthy children aged 2 to 11 years—Position of ADA." *Journal of the American Dietetics Association*. January 1999

Connor, WE, and Connor, SL. "The case for a low-fat, high-carbohydrate diet." *The New England Journal of Medicine*. August 1997

Cross, A, et al. "Snacking patterns among 1,800 adults and children." *Journal of the American Dietetic Association*. December 1994

Epstein, L. "Methodological Issues and Ten-Year Outcomes for Obese Children." *Prevention and Treatment of Childhood Obesity*. The New York Academy of Sciences, New York. 1993

Hammer, LD. "The development of eating behavior in childhood." *Pediatric Clinics of North America*. June 1992

Johnson, S, and Birch, L. "Parents' and children's adiposity and eating style." *Pediatrics*. November 1994

Klesges, RC. "Parental influence on food selection in young children and its relationship to childhood obesity." *American Journal of Clinical Nutrition*. April 1991

Kosharek, S. *If Your Child Is Overweight*. The American Dietetic Association. 1993

Lin, BH, et al. "The diets of America's children: influences of dining out, household characteristics, and nutrition knowledge. *U.S. Department of Agriculture Economic Report Number 746*. December 1996

Ludwig, DS, et al. "Relation between consumption of sugar-sweetened drinks and childhood obesity: a prospective, observational analysis. *The Lancet*. February 2001

Nicklas, T, et al. "Breakfast consumption affects adequacy of total daily intake in children." *Journal of the American Dietetic Association*. August 1993

Obarzanek, E, et al. "Safety of a fat-reduced diet: the dietary intervention study in children. *Pediatrics*. July 1997

Pennington, J. *Bowes & Church's Food Values of Portions Commonly Used*. Lippincott, Williams & Williams. 1998

Satter, EM. "Internal regulation and evolution of normal growth as the basis for prevention of obesity in children." *Journal of the American Dietetic Association*. September 1996

U.S. Department of Agriculture, Human Nutrition Information Service. *Food Guide Pyramid*. August 1992

U.S. Food and Drug Administration. *The Food Label*. May 1999

Part IV. Focus on Fitness

American Academy of Pediatrics. "Television and the Family." 2000

Andersen, RE, et al. "Relationship of physical activity and television watching with body weight and level of fatness among children." *Journal of the American Medical Association*. March 1998

Borra, ST, et al. "Food, physical activity, and fun: inspiring America's kids to more healthful lifestyles." *Journal of the American Dietetic Association*. July 1995

Elder, JP, et al. "Direct home observation of the promoting of physical activity in sedentary and active Mexican- and Anglo-American children." *Journal of Developmental and Behavioral Pediatrics*. February 1998

Epstein, L, et al. "Effects of decreasing sedentary behavior and increasing activity on weight change in obese children." *Health Psychology*. March 1995

Ferguson, K, et al. "Attitudes, knowledge and beliefs as predictors of exercise intent and behavior in schoolchildren." *Journal of School Health*. March 1989

Fogelholm, M, et al. "Parent-child relationship of physical activity patterns and obesity." *International Journal of Obesity Related Metabolic Disorders*. December 1999

Gortmaker, SL, et al. "Television viewing as a cause of increasing obesity among children in the United States, 1986–1990." *Archives of Pediatric and Adolescent Medicine.* April 1996

International Life Science Institute. "A survey of parents and children about physical activity patterns." July 1997

Nader, PR, et al. "The effect of adult participation in a school-based family intervention to improve children's diet and physical activity: the child and adolescent trial for cardiovascular health." *Preventive Medicine.* July–August 1996

Pender, NJ. "Motivation for physical activity among children and adolescents." *Annual Review of Nursing Research.* 1998

Robinson, TN. "Reducing children's television viewing to prevent obesity: a randomized controlled trial. *Journal of the American Medical Association.* October 1999

Sothern, MS, et al. "Motivating the obese child to move: the role of structured exercise in pediatric weight management. *Southern Medical Journal.* June 1999

Stone, EJ, et al. "Effects of physical activity interventions in youth: review and synthesis." *American Journal of Preventive Medicine.* November 1998

Part V. Facilitate Change

Abramovitz, BA, and Birch LL. "Five-year-old girls' ideas about dieting are predicted by their mothers' dieting." *Journal of the American Dietetic Association.* October 2000

American Dietetic Association. "Position of the American Dietetic Association: nutrition intervention in the treatment of anorexia nervosa, bulimia nervosa, and binge eating." *Journal of the American Dietetic Association.* August 1994

Berg, F. "Eating disorders affect both the mind and body." *Healthy Weight Journal.* March/April 1995

Davison, KK, and Birch, LL. "Weight status, parent reaction, and self-concept in five-year-old girls." *Pediatrics.* January 2001

Ikeda, J, and Naworski, P. *Am I Fat? Helping Young Children Accept Differences in Body Size.* ETR Associates, Santa Cruz, CA. 1992

Johnson, C. "Raising largely positive kids." *Obesity and Health.* November–December 1993

Kolody, B, and Sallis, JF. "A prospective study of ponderosity, body image, self-concept, and psychological variables in children." *Journal of Developmental and Behavioral Pediatrics*. February 1995

Kristian von Almen, T, et al. "Psychosocial Considerations in the Treatment of Childhood Obesity." *The Obese Child*. Karger, Basel, Switzerland: Pediatric Adolescent Medicine. 1992

Leon, GR, et al. "Personality and behavioral vulnerabilities associated with risk status for eating disorders in adolescent girls." *Journal of Abnormal Psychology*. August 1993

Pierce, JW. "Self-esteem, parental appraisal and body size in children." *Journal of Child Psychology and Psychiatry*. October 1993

Schreiber, GB, et al. "Weight modification efforts reported by black and white preadolescent girls: National Heart, Lung, and Blood Institute Growth and Health Study. *Pediatrics*. July 1996

Index